The Multiple Sclerosis Companion

Anke Friedrich

The Multiple Sclerosis Companion

Answers to the most frequently asked
questions from people with MS

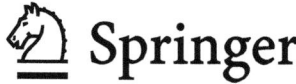 Springer

Anke Friedrich
Zentrum für ambulante Neurologie
Essen, Germany

ISBN 978-3-662-67539-7   ISBN 978-3-662-67540-3   (eBook)
https://doi.org/10.1007/978-3-662-67540-3

Preface

Maintaining autonomy with a chronic disease and having a meaningful say in therapeutic decisions or supporting and accompanying an affected person require knowledge. Although there is a wealth of information on the internet, many of those affected and their relatives are rather confused by it. The fact is that there is an immense need for information.

After patient events, I am regularly asked: "Do you have a script for this?," "Can I read about it somewhere?" or "Can I also do something myself?"

I have attempted to fulfil these wishes and am very pleased to be able to present this book to you. It is the answer to the most frequently asked questions of MS patients and their relatives, which are asked again and again in daily practice and cannot be answered to this extent and with this clarity in everyday consultations due to lack of time.

This companion consists of three parts. In Parts I and II, you will find comprehensive information about the disease, how it is detected and how it is treated, so that you as a person affected can use this knowledge to make therapeutic decisions together with your neurologist or, as a family member, to develop an understanding of the disease and therapy.

In Part III, you will receive very interesting new information on the topics of nutrition, intestine, immune system and MS. Here, I would like to motivate all patients to also integrate supplementary measures into their lives in order to additionally improve their quality of life and well-being. I am happy if my MS companion becomes a valuable and informative guide for you, enabling you to actively shape your life.

Essen, Germany   Anke Friedrich
Autumn 2022

Acknowledgements

First of all, I would like to thank all the MS patients who have come to see me in the consultation hours and for allowing me to experience the disease, the associated worries, many questions and also the solutions and perspectives over many years. Thanks to all those patients who inspired me to write this book by asking me those many questions and also to those of you abroad for encouraging me to put this book into English.

Thank you Jennifer for letting me share your story, which was the final kick for the idea of this MS Companion.

A very special thank you to Shayne Drury. You penned the wonderful drawings that make the book vivid and alive. Thank you for your great support and encouragement when I got "stuck" or had doubts and for your patience with me on this book project over the last few years.

Many thanks especially to Verena, eagle eye, a technical miracle, for always being there when things were "on fire". To my brother and my friends who read and corrected the manuscript drafts, kept asking questions and gave me lots of suggestions, helped me with various technical problems and enriched the book with photographic processing and recipe ideas. Jens, Martina, Katrin, Iris and Angela—thank you for your great support.

I would like to thank Katja Seng, MD. Thank you very much dear Katja, for allowing me to benefit from your great radiological knowledge and for letting me use the MRI images.

And I thank my patients E. and A. for allowing me to tell their medical stories in this publication. It is my privilege and pleasure to be your neurologist.

Furthermore, my heartfelt thanks go to Dr. Christine Lerche, Senior Editor, Programmplanung Medizin, Book and ePublishing at Springer Verlag, who believed in my concept and intensively accompanied and supported me as an author. I would also very much like to thank Sylvana Freyberg, PhD, Senior Editor, Medicine Books, Continental Europe and the UK at Springer, for making this book in English possible. Without you and your help here, the English version would never have happened!

Thanks also to the team at Springer Verlag, for their professionalism and friendly competence along the way.

And a very special thank you also goes to my editor, Dr. med. Martina Kahl-Scholz, who professionally and reliably assisted me in the final phase and took my often unwieldy medical language and jargon and made it easy to understand for non-medical people.

Thank you Shayne once again for all your help in putting this book into English. I would never have managed the English version without you!

I have had the privilege of working with a super team and great colleagues in our practice, the "Zentrum für ambulante Neurologie" in Essen, Germany, for many years—I thank you all very much for that too.

And I thank my parents for their loving support my whole life long. As doctors themselves, they led the way and encouraged my enthusiasm for medicine.

Last but not least, of course, a very big thank you to you, the readers, who bought this MS Companion.

Contents

Part II   MS: Understanding the Therapy

6   How MS Is Treated

7   What To Do in an Acute MS Attack

8   I'm Fine: Why Therapy?

9   MS Therapy Yesterday and Today

About the Author

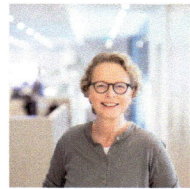

Anke Friedrich, born in 1964 in Duisburg-Rheinhausen, grew up in Geldern on the Lower Rhine and studied medicine at Heinrich Heine University in Düsseldorf, where she obtained her doctorate in paediatric haematology and oncology in 1991. After working for 2 years as an internist in Brig/Switzerland and in oncology in Duisburg-Rheinhausen, her interest in neurological disease patterns grew, so that her further training path led via neurology (Oberhausen), neurosurgery (University Hospital Essen) and psychiatry (LVR Hospital Essen) to become a specialist in neurology. In 1998 she decided to become self-employed and joined a group practice in Essen where she has played a decisive role over the last 25 years in developing the "Zentrum für ambulante Neurologie". Her conviction of a holistic concept of health also led her to Traditional Chinese Medicine (TCM) with acupuncture training (Beijing/China and Bramsche/Germany). Her experience that the environment and the space also have an influence on the health and well-being of people also led Dr. Friedrich to train as a Feng Shui and Geomancy consultant. During her many years of neurological practice, she became particularly interested in the treatment and support of patients with MS, and over the years Multiple Sclerosis has become her main area of practice. She is a sought-after speaker on this topic, gives specialist lectures for medical colleagues and "MS nurses" and knows the concerns and questions of MS sufferers first-hand. Inspired by these questions and the desire for more information, the idea for her now published *Multiple Sclerosis Companion* came about. Anke Friedrich lives in Essen, is married and in her free time enjoys photography and cycling in the countryside. She is interested in architecture, design and art and loves spending time together with her family, dogs and friends over a delicious meal and a good glass of red wine.

Part I

MS: Understanding the Disease

1

What Is MS? A First Overview

1.1 Jennifer's Story

In spring 2016, a concerned friend called me from London. A lame leg for several months, tingling in the hands every now and then, an MRI of the head "with white spots" and the suspected diagnosis of multiple sclerosis were her reasons for calling. This friend had just turned 60 at the time, and even though this age is not quite typical for the initial diagnosis of MS, it really had to be considered with these symptoms. Further clarification including a cerebrospinal fluid examination confirmed the suspicion, and Jennifer had been discharged from hospital with the diagnosis and a host of unanswered questions. She asked me—as almost all sufferers do—the question: "Is there anything I can do myself?" Indeed, she can! And in our long telephone conversation, I tried to shed light on her darkness.

It was over a year before I met Jennifer again at a family party in London in the summer of 2017. She was full of energy and looked her best. Jennifer told me how much my information had helped her to cope with her chronic illness. While she had initially been discharged from hospital feeling powerless and with the inner conviction that her active life was now over, my information had motivated her and given her back the feeling that she could also do something herself. She was especially helped by my nutritional advice and the fact that I could tell her about some of my very sporty MS patients who are marathon runners. Inspired and motivated by this, she had changed her diet and resumed her sporting goal of a trans-European tour. Her big passion is cycling, and so she crossed Europe—from west to east with her bike

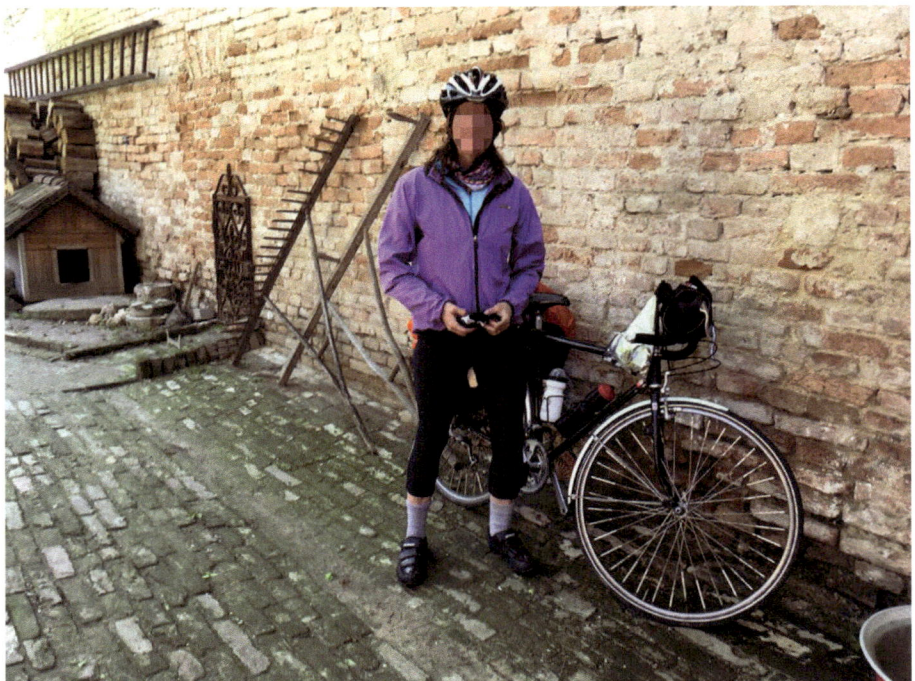

Fig. 1.1 Jennifer on her way

(Fig. 1.1)—a European tour from the west coast of Ireland to Constanta on the Black Sea in Romania. In several stages, she covered a total of 5200 km!

After our meeting at the aforementioned family festival, a week of relaxation followed for me in Andalusia. With temperatures well over 35°C, I spent a lot of time under a large, old, shady walnut tree (Fig. 1.2) by the pool of the small, secluded finca. I thought about our conversation in London and realised how important it is, especially for people with chronic illnesses, to maintain autonomy. How often does it happen in everyday practice that patients like Jennifer are discharged from hospital after being diagnosed with MS and are looking for answers to their many questions? And how often have I been asked: What else can I do myself?

In the beginning, therefore, there is information. Without knowledge, it is not possible to have a say in therapeutic decisions.

It is equally important to create motivation and perspective.

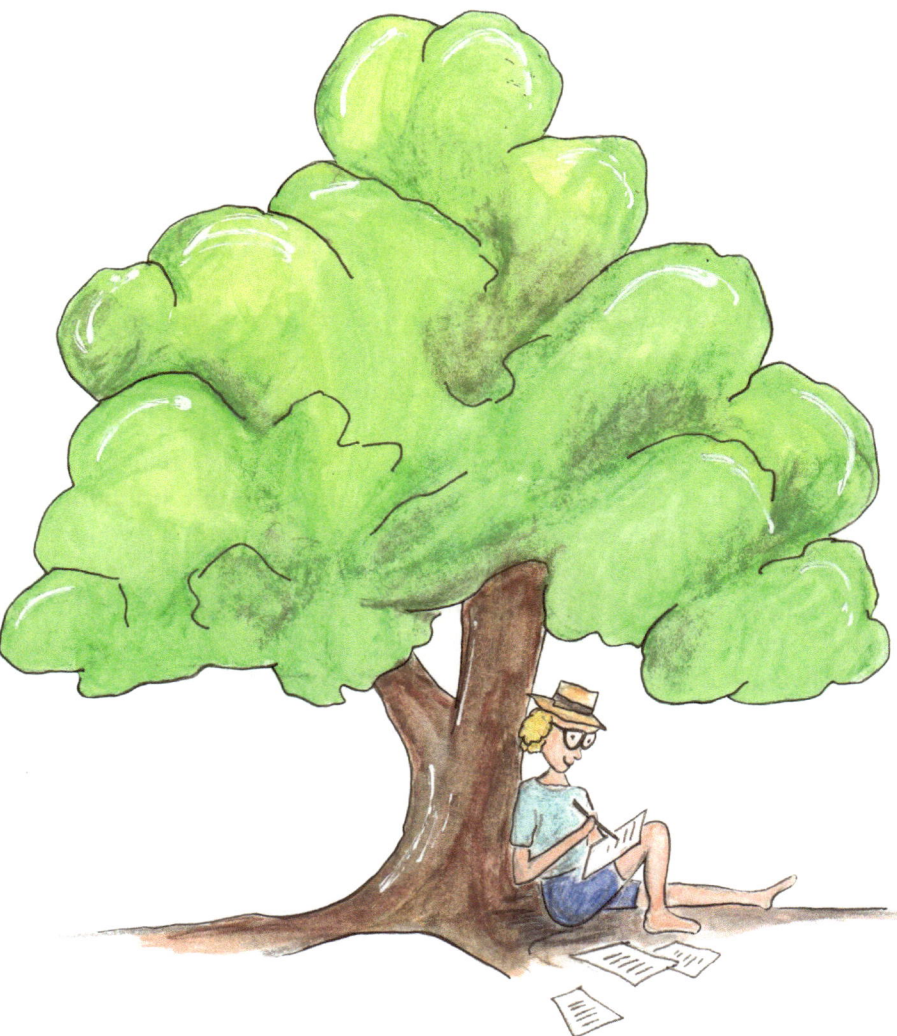

Fig. 1.2   Under the old walnut tree

After Jennifer's story, I knew that if I could motivate **one** person through this information to become active again in living with a chronic illness, I could reach even **more** people through a book. And so, I started writing.

Jennifer's story is an individual one, but she is not an isolated case. In the following chapter, let us first look at some figures about multiple sclerosis.

1.2   First Things First: A Few Facts and Figures About MS

When a young person is confronted with a suspected diagnosis of MS, their world often collapses at first. "Will I end up in a wheelchair?", "Can I ever start a family?", "What about my job?", "What happens now?"—all these thoughts and more run through their minds at the same time. At that moment, all thinking freezes, and the doctor's explanatory words can hardly be taken in. This is why, according to my experience, several short-term revisits to the practice are important after the diagnosis has been established. Only through repeat appointments with "tidbits of information" does light gradually come into the darkness.

Even though many people have never heard of MS before and may not know anyone with MS, MS is the **most common chronic inflammatory disease of the central nervous system in young adulthood**. So, you are not alone with your disease. In Germany, more than 240,000 people are affected, in the UK approximately 130,000 are affected, in Europe the number is around 1 million people and worldwide there are approximately 2.5 million people living with MS. MS sufferers are usually between 20 and 40 years old at the time of diagnosis and therefore still have their lives ahead of them. About 5% even become ill before the age of 16. MS particularly affects young women, as over 70% of all MS patients are female.

When MS symptoms first appear, they can be misinterpreted. This is because sometimes typical symptoms flash up here and there for a few days and then slowly recede, are then forgotten about and come back after months or possibly only after years in a completely different place. This is precisely the reason why the disease is sometimes only recognised after a delay.

The number of people with MS has almost doubled over the last 20–25 years not only in Germany where I live, but also across much of the Western world. What could be the reasons? If one takes into account the distribution of MS disease worldwide, there is a particular accumulation between the 44th and 64th northern latitude. The greater the distance from the equator, the greater the risk of disease. This applies to both the northern and southern hemispheres. Why is this so?

According to data from the World Health Organization (WHO), the UK, Europe and North America are particularly affected. Broken down by income, there is a clustering of the richer income strata of the affected countries. What could be the reasons? How do these regions differ? Is it genetic differences, e.g. in our innate immune system? Is it environmental factors, such as childhood infections? Or are they different diets? Is it different light conditions with different sun intensity? Are there lifestyle factors that affect our immune system which play an essential role in MS?

These interesting questions are currently the focus of many scientific studies. Since there are indications from studies on twins that genetics is only about 30% causal for the onset of the disease and the rest of 70% can be attributed to the environment, it is worthwhile taking a closer look at these environmental factors (see Part III).

Even though the actual cause of MS development is still not clear, there have been many new insights into the immune system and its changes in MS, especially in recent years. This knowledge is also increasing the therapeutic possibilities to treat MS.

1.3 How the Central Nervous System Is Structured: Anatomy

MS is a chronic inflammatory disease of the central nervous system (CNS). To understand this better, let us first take a quick trip into the anatomy of the nervous system (Fig. 1.3).

1.3.1 The Central Nervous System: Brain and Spinal Cord

The central nervous system is composed of the brain and the spinal cord. The brain is the "control centre", while the spinal cord is a huge "cable channel" that connects the brain with the periphery, i.e. the rest of the body, so that information can be passed from the brain right down to the end of the baby toe or finger and back to the brain again.

The anatomical areas of the brain important to us in this book are the cerebrum, the corpus callosum, the cerebellum and the brainstem, which then passes into the spinal cord (Fig. 1.4).

1.3.2 Corpus Callosum and Spinal Cord

In MS, the corpus callosum and the spinal cord are important anatomical structures to pay special attention to. The corpus callosum consists of nerve

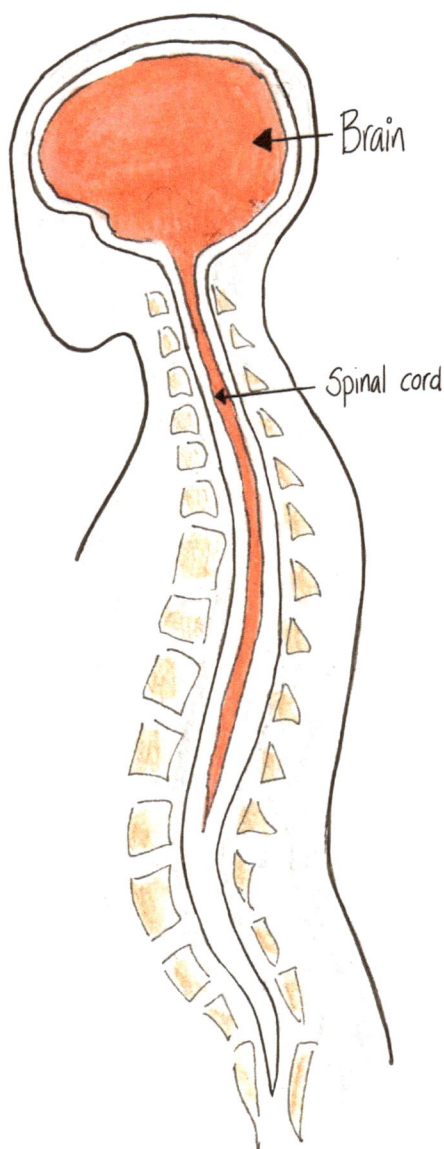

Fig. 1.3 The central nervous system (CNS) with brain and spinal cord shown in red

fibres that connect both halves of the brain. **Inflammatory changes in** the corpus callosum and also in the spinal cord are very typical of MS disease.

The spinal cord as an extension of the brainstem can also be affected by these inflammations, and it runs protected and surrounded by the vertebral bodies in the so-called spinal canal. As the cervical medulla, it runs through

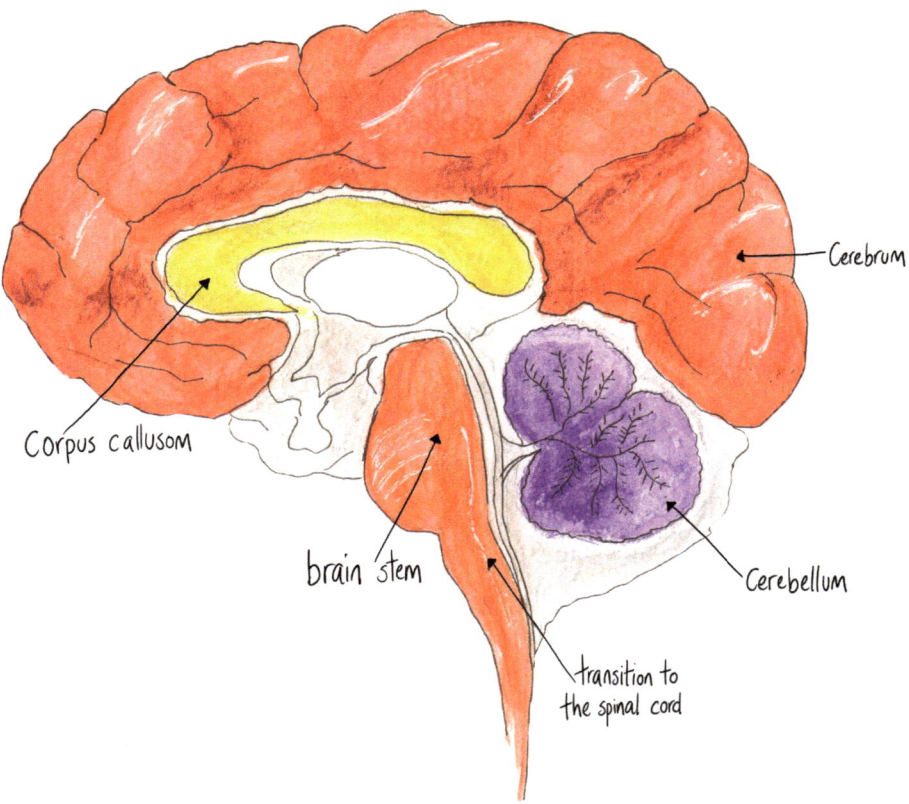

Fig. 1.4 Cerebrum, cerebellum, corpus callosum, brainstem, transition to spinal cord

the cervical spine and as the thoracic medulla through the thoracic spine. The spinal cord ends at the first lumbar vertebral body of the lumbar spine. The lumbar spine therefore **no** longer contains a spinal cord.

Since MS only affects the central nervous system (CNS), typical MS changes can only be found up to or above the first lumbar vertebra.

1.4   Immune System and its Influence on the Central Nervous System: The Consequences

The immune system is such a complex system that we still do not understand it in its entirety. Even if the actual cause of the development of MS is not yet clear, there is more and more knowledge about the changes in the immune system in MS.

1.4.1   When the Body Attacks Itself: Autoimmune Disease

MS is an autoimmune disease. This generic term refers to diseases in which the immune system is directed against structures of the patient's own body. In MS, the body's own immune system is directed against certain protein components of the central nervous system. The body's own blood cells, the so-called lymphocytes, attack the body's own structures as if they were an enemy. Lymphocytes are suddenly able to overcome the "blood–brain barrier"—a barrier that exists between the blood and the brain and which actually forms a barrier for such cells—and migrate into the central nervous system. Once in the brain, they set off further inflammatory reactions and ultimately destroy

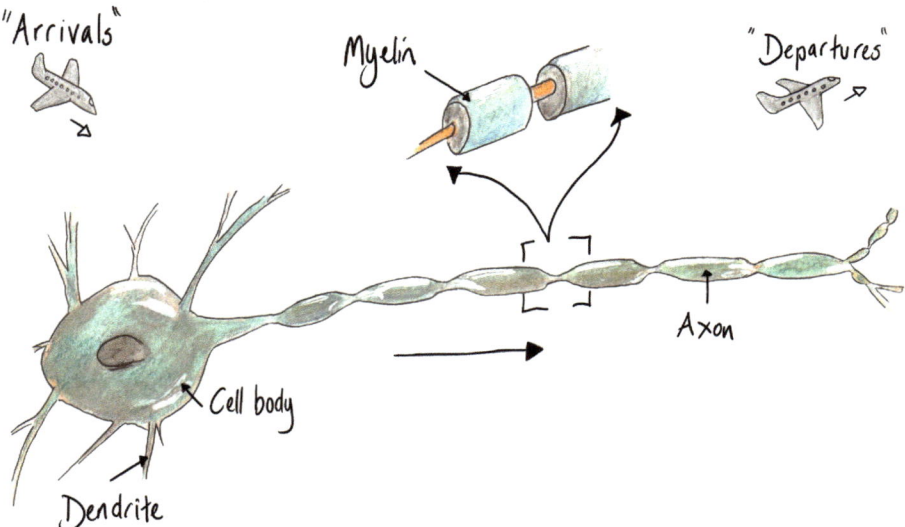

Fig. 1.5   The healthy nerve cell

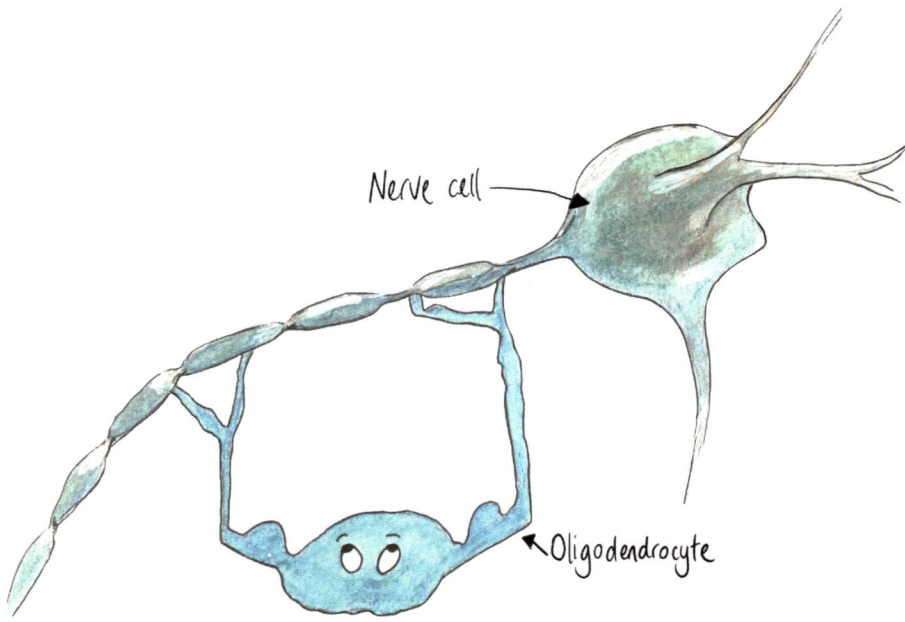

Fig. 1.6   The myelin-producing oligodendrocyte at work

nerve cells. To get a better idea of the damage caused by the autoimmune process, let us first have a look at the anatomy of a healthy nerve cell (Fig. 1.5).

1.4.2   Nerve Cell: Dendrites, Axon and its Sheath, the Myelin

A nerve cell consists of a cell body with very many small "arms" and one long arm. The small arms are called "dendrites". They conduct information from other cells to the cell body of the nerve cell. The dendrites thus correspond to the "arrival" at the airport, so to speak. The long arm of the nerve cell is called the axon. The axon is the outgoing cable, quasi-"departure", which passes the information away from the cell body on to the next cell (see also Fig. 1.5).

Axons are sheathed in an insulating layer called myelin, which in turn consists of fats and proteins. The myelin is formed in the central nervous system by special cells called oligodendrocytes. Through the myelin sheathing, the oligodendrocytes protect and support the nerve cell and also serve as an energy supplier for the nerve cell (Fig. 1.6).

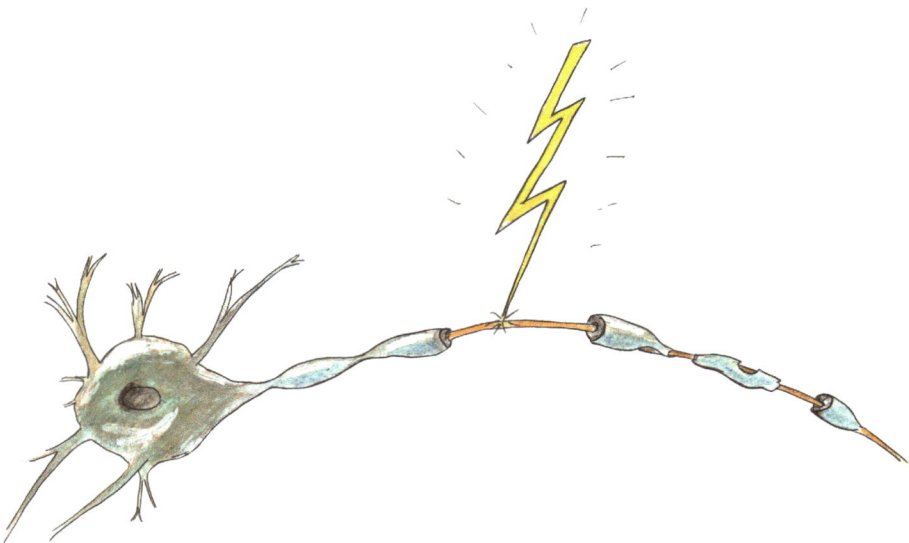

Fig. 1.7 The damaged insulation of a nerve cell

1.4.3 Short Circuit in the Nervous System and Its Consequences

You can imagine an axon simplified like an electric cable. Inside is the wire and around it the sheath for insulation. This sheath corresponds to the myelin, which is responsible for the speed of impulse transmission.

> The thicker the myelin sheathing, the faster the conduction speed of the nerve cell and thus the transmission of information.

Nerve cells with a thick myelin layer therefore run much faster than thinly myelinated nerve cells. Just as the electrical cable can short-circuit if the insulation is damaged, the axon slows down the transport of information if the myelin is damaged—and this is exactly what happens in MS.

This is because the inflammatory attack in MS is directed against the myelin. The insulating layer is damaged, which is called "demyelination". Demyelination of the cable leads to a slowing down of the information transport and subsequently to symptoms of disease (Fig. 1.7).

The autoimmune inflammatory process is initially only directed against the myelin, but in the further course, cell damage can also occur, so that the axon also perishes. The consequence is a loss of the entire nerve cell. Over the years, increasing nerve cell loss ultimately leads to a loss of brain substance or volume (brain atrophy). Scars form, and just like scars on the skin, they do not have the same texture as healthy tissue. The scarred healing is harder and more rigid (and is also called "sclerosis"). This gives the disease its name because **multiple sclerosis** means **many hardenings**. More detailed information on the immune process in MS can be found in Chap. 3, "A Trip into Our Immune System".

1.4.4   Iceberg Model: Disease Activity and Inflammatory Activity

The consequence of this inflammatory reaction and the associated demyelination of the nerve cells is neurological deficits—typical symptoms of MS. These can vary greatly depending on the location and size of the single inflammatory lesions. Since the single inflammatory lesions in the brain are often very small, it is usually difficult to assign the clear localisation to the disease symptoms and vice versa. It also happens that inflammatory processes in the brain are not even perceived by the MS sufferer, i.e. they run "silently", which is then referred to as "subclinical" in medical jargon. For example, in 50–70% of patients with

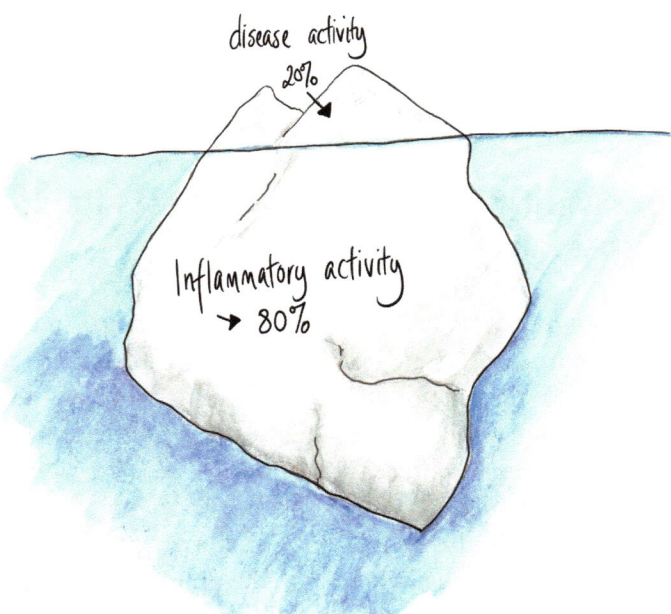

Fig. 1.8   Disease activity and inflammatory activity

visual impairment due to optic nerve inflammation, other inflammatory lesions can be detected in the brain, but these have not yet led to symptoms. For this reason, if you have optic neuritis, then an MRI of the brain is necessary (more on this in Chap. 4), in order to look for further subclinical lesions.

It is therefore important to distinguish between disease activity (what really shows up in symptoms) and inflammatory activity (what tissue is actually already changed/damaged by inflammation), because only a small part (approx. 20%) shows up in the form of clinical symptoms as "disease activity". However, much more happens "under the surface in secret" as subclinical inflammatory activity (approx. 80%).

The "iceberg model" illustrates this situation. The small peak visible above the surface corresponds to the disease activity with symptoms, while the much larger part lies hidden and symbolises the subclinical "inflammatory activity" (Fig. 1.8).

> Any inflammatory change in the brain, however—whether it leads to symptoms or not—should be taken equally seriously because it indicates disease progression and can eventually lead to brain changes in the form of scarring and brain volume loss.

The described autoimmune process and the associated demyelination with nerve cell destruction should be recognised as soon as possible.

> The earlier the disease can be intervened in, the sooner the consequential damage can be prevented.

1.5 How Multiple Sclerosis Manifests Itself: MS Relapse and Typical Symptoms

What is an MS relapse and what are typical MS symptoms? An MS relapse is defined as the occurrence of new symptoms attributable to the central nervous system that last longer than 24 h and are not related to a febrile infection. In most cases, relapsing symptoms develop over several hours to days, last for a few days to weeks and then slowly subside.

The **symptom**(s) are caused by the "inflammatory attack" and the associated tissue swelling in the affected region of the brain and spinal cord. If the inflammation recedes and the swelling goes down, the symptoms slowly disappear—but not always completely. If the inflammatory attack causes extensive cell damage with scarring, residual symptoms may remain.

1.5.1 "Typical" MS Symptoms

The MS symptoms depend on the location of the inflammatory attack in the central nervous system. Although there is hardly a symptom that cannot occur in MS, there are some particularly "typical MS symptoms". Typical initial symptoms that should make you think of MS are above all the following:

1. Blurred, "milky" discoloured vision due to optic nerve inflammation. Often, the visual disorder is associated with pain when the eye moves (so-called movement pain).
2. Tingling, sensory disturbances or numbness in different parts of the body, especially rising from the feet and/or the hands.
3. Weakness and lack of strength in the legs and/or arms, sometimes associated with bladder problems.
4. Balance disorders, dizziness and gait unsteadiness.

All the symptoms described above can of course also occur in combination.

To illustrate how vision changes with optic neuritis, look at the following picture with our two dogs Chico and Grace (Fig. 1.9).

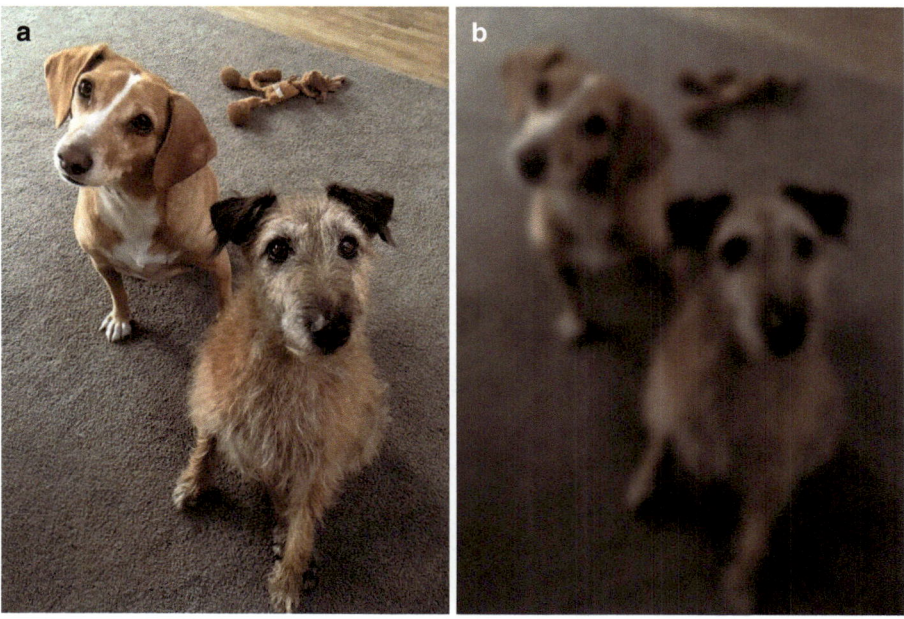

Fig. 1.9 **(a)** Normal vision. **(b)** Visual disturbance with optic nerve inflammation

While the image on the left represents sharp normal vision, on the right, you see Chico and Grace blurred and less colourful. This or similar is how a person with optic neuritis sees.

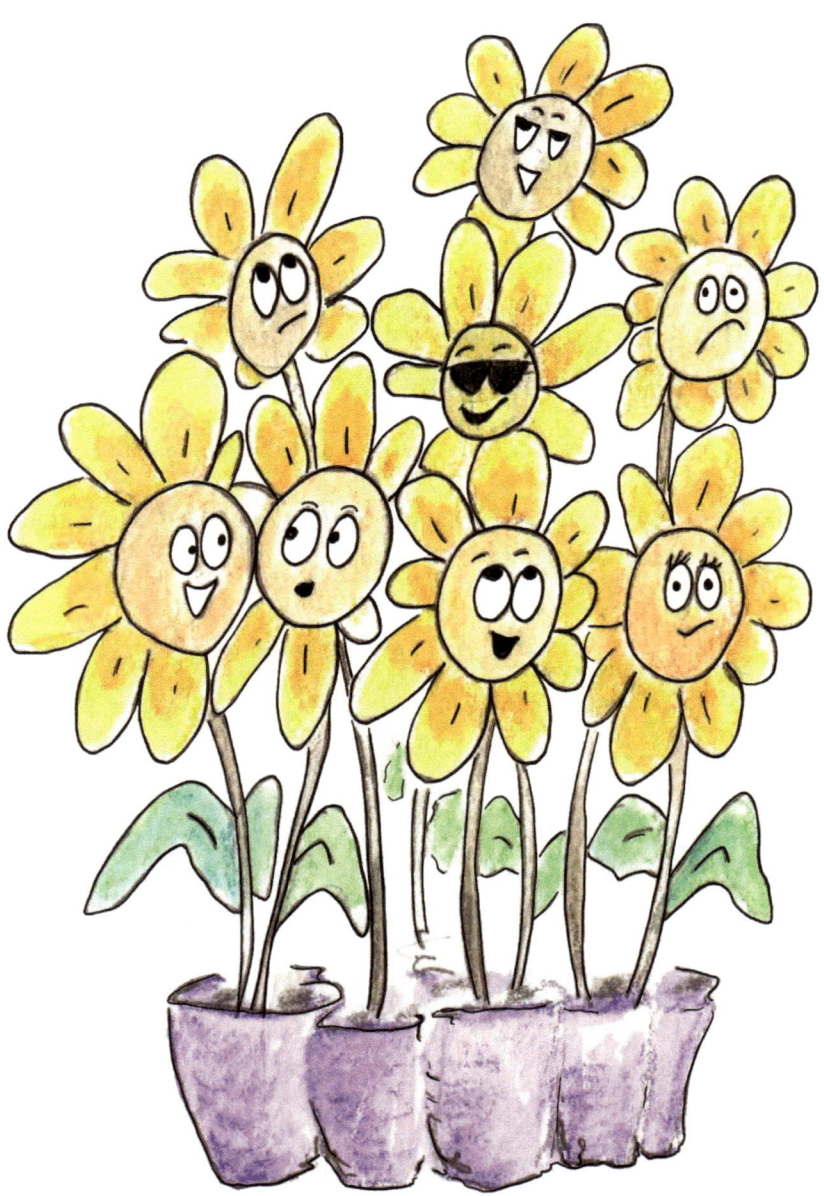

Fig. 1.10 MS—the disease with many faces

1.5.2   MS Can Be Overlooked at First

Since MS symptoms do not usually develop acutely—i.e. from one moment to the next—but rather more slowly over hours or days, and can also disappear on their own, some people with MS do not consult a doctor at all when they first experience symptoms. That is why it is important to ask specifically about past symptoms when taking the patient's medical history. Because the first symptoms of the disease are often not recognised as such, the diagnosis can be delayed.

1.6   How the Disease Can Run Its Course

Not only because of the many different symptoms, but also because of the very different courses of the disease, MS is rightly called "the disease with many faces" (Fig. 1.10).

Especially at the beginning of the disease, most people with MS experience relapses, which means that symptoms develop and often disappear completely. In some patients, the relapses occur very frequently, and in others with long intervals of sometimes several years. This initial relapsing-remitting course is the most common, accounting for about 85% of all MS patients, and is called "relapsing-remitting MS" (**RRMS**), regardless of the frequency of relapses. A relapsing-remitting course can occur with or without residual symptoms.

In the further course of the disease, however, symptoms can also gradually worsen after the initial relapsing symptoms and thus cause restrictions. This course of the disease is referred to as "secondary progressive MS" (**SPMS**). Transitions between the individual forms of progression are also possible, e.g. "secondary progressive with onset relapses".

Rarely, there are courses of the disease without relapses, but these also exist. In this case, there is a continuous, slow deterioration from the beginning with increasing disability. This course is called "primary progressive MS" (**PPMS**) and occurs in less than 10% of all MS cases. This rare form of progression is to be regarded as a special form, because experience has shown that it does not respond so well to the usual MS therapies.

After this first overview of MS, in the next chapter "Do I Really Have MS?", we will look at the path to diagnosis and the necessary examinations.

2

Do I Really Have MS?

2.1 The Path to Diagnosis

In this chapter, we look at what conditions must be met in order to make the diagnosis of MS. Multiple sclerosis is characterised on the one hand, as the name "multiple" suggests, by the detection of **multiple** changes in the central nervous system. Secondly, it is a relapsing disease, i.e. recurring symptoms over **time**. And with that, we already have the two essential diagnostic criteria of MS. This is called "spatial and dissemination in time", which I would like to explain in more detail below.

2.1.1 Important Diagnostic Criteria: Spatial and Dissemination in Time

Dissemination is derived from the Latin "disseminare", which means "to sow". Dissemination means "sowing" or also "scattering, distribution".

> "Dissemination in space" or also "spatial distribution" means that typical inflammatory lesions must be detected at several locations in the central nervous system for the diagnosis.

Spatial dissemination is often abbreviated in the literature to "dissemination in space" (DIS), i.e. the occurrence of pathological changes in more than one place. Thus, it is not enough to detect only one lesion to diagnose MS. The characteristic of MS is that inflammatory lesions must be present at several typical sites in the CNS.

In addition to dissemination in space, the criterion of "dissemination in time" (DIT) must also be fulfilled before the diagnosis of MS can be made.

> "Dissemination in time" means that disease activity must occur at different times.

The relapsing course and thus the recurrent occurrence of disease activity form the second essential characteristic of MS disease. The proof of this dissemination in time can be provided either by several but at least two clinical relapses or by the proof of lesions of different ages in the MRI. Dissemination over time is often abbreviated in the literature to "DIT" as "dissemination in time".

> In order to diagnose MS, both characteristics of the disease, i.e. the criteria of spatial and dissemination in time, must be fulfilled. And that is not all. In addition, other diseases that can cause similar symptoms must be excluded by blood and cerebrospinal fluid examination (lumbar puncture).

The investigation methods that are necessary to detect spatial and dissemination in time (DIS and DIT) are explained below.

2.2   What Tests Are Used to Detect MS: Methods

As you have already heard, inflammatory MS changes can develop in the brain or spinal cord without causing any symptoms. Therefore, a distinction must be made between disease activity and inflammatory activity, which is best illustrated by the iceberg model (Sect. 1.4). The inflammatory activity below the surface is much higher (80%) than the actual disease activity (20%), which manifests itself as a clinical episode. Therefore, the inflammatory activity under the surface must be specifically searched for. The neurologist needs:

1. The exact **anamnesis**, i.e. the medical history
2. The **neurological examination**
3. The additional electrical examinations with the "**evoked potentials**" (**EP**)
4. The **MRI** (MRI skull, cervical and thoracic spine)

5. **Blood and cerebrospinal fluid examination** (= lumbar puncture, LP abbreviated)

2.2.1 Questions About Questions: What the Anamnesis Can Do

First of all, the current symptoms are asked about during the anamnesis. Just by describing the symptoms, the neurologist can obtain clues as to whether the symptoms can be traced back to one or several places of origin. For example, if a patient complains of a new visual disturbance with additional numbness in the leg, these two symptoms cannot be anatomically assigned to a single site of origin in the central nervous system and would thus already be a first indication of a multifocal (i.e. found in several places) disease (criterion of dissemination in space). The dissemination in time can sometimes also be inferred to from the medical history, namely if MS-suspicious symptoms have already occurred in the past. If one asks specifically, clues from the past often emerge. Sometimes, these symptoms are not actively remembered because they may have spontaneously disappeared. That is why it is important to ask specifically about them. In this way, even a detailed anamnesis can provide a first indication of a **multifocal** and **multi-period** disease.

2.2.2 When Your Doctor Swings the Hammer: The Neurological Examination

The neurological examination serves to detect neurological deficits and to draw conclusions about the place of origin of the damage. The distribution and spread of the neurological abnormalities provide the neurologist with information as to whether the symptoms can be assigned to the **central nervous system.** It is also often possible to determine in this way whether the neurological abnormalities originate from one or more sites (dissemination in space).

2.2.3 Measuring the "Cable Run" Electrically: The "EPs"

The additional electrical examinations, the so-called evoked potentials (EPs), offer a possibility to identify further sites of damage (dissemination in space). In these examinations, the "cables" in the central nervous system are measured. The values of potential amplitudes and conduction times in milliseconds (ms) are determined in a side-by-side comparison, which provide possible indications of damage "in the cable". This technique is particularly important for examining the visual pathway and identifying possible spinal cord lesions.

As an example, the so-called visual evoked potential (VEP) is described here. The VEP is used to assess the optic nerve. The person being examined looks at a screen with a chessboard-like pattern in which black-and-white fields constantly change; this creates repeated visual impressions on the retina of the eye, which are transmitted as nerve impulses to the visual cortex and can be recorded by electrodes on the scalp. A delay in the averaged potentials gives an indication of the presence of damage in the cable course of the optic nerve. In a similar way, "other cables", for example the long nerve tracts in the spinal cord, can also be measured.

2.2.4   For the Earliest Possible Detection: The MRI

The magnetic resonance imaging (MRI) plays a central role in MS diagnosis. It shows inflammatory lesions at different locations in the brain, dissemination in space (DIS), and under special circumstances, it can help to distinguish between old and new inflammatory lesions and thus provide evidence of the dissemination in time (DIT). The distinction can be made by administering contrast agent (gadolinium). New lesions show gadolinium enhancements only up to 3 months, and after this period of time, you cannot see any effect of the contrast agent in the lesions anymore.

If you find new and old lesions side by side in the first MRI, this shows that they came at different times and therefore the criteria for dissemination in time are fulfilled. In this way, the diagnosis can be made early with an MRI, often **before** a second clinical relapse event occurs. Since the MRI is very important for MS diagnosis and follow-up, I will come back to this in a detailed MRI chapter later on (Chap. 4: Why MRI?).

2.2.5   More Than Just Water: CSF Examination
and Oligoclonal Bands

With the purpose of diagnosing MS, and in addition to proof of spatial and dissemination in time, "other diseases" that can trigger MS-like symptoms must be ruled out. These include, for example, Lyme disease, a tick-borne disease, or vasculitis, an inflammatory disease of the blood vessels. In order to distinguish such diseases from MS, a blood and cerebrospinal fluid (CSF) test is carried out.

Since blood and CSF are separate areas due to the blood–brain barrier, the blood examination does **not** replace the CSF examination. To obtain cerebrospinal fluid, a so-called lumbar puncture is carried out. The cerebrospinal fluid (CSF) is the fluid that flows around the brain and the spinal cord, thus hydraulically protecting it against knocks. The cerebrospinal fluid is located in a designated space, the dural space, which is surrounded by a sheath—the dura. The dura is the "hard brain skin" that provides additional protection for the delicate CNS. While the spinal cord, as described in Chap. 1, ends at the level of the first lumbar vertebra, the dura extends even further down to the first sacral vertebra as a so-called dural sac, which is also filled with cerebrospinal fluid there. The cerebrospinal fluid is taken from the lumbar region between the third and fourth or fourth and fifth lumbar vertebrae with the help of a fine needle and then examined.

Due to the spatial proximity of the CNS and the cerebrospinal fluid, the examination of the cerebrospinal fluid allows conclusions to be drawn about diseases of the brain and spinal cord. However, the lumbar puncture is used to not only exclude other diseases, but also detect autoimmune inflammatory changes in the cerebrospinal fluid that are suspicious for MS. The so-called oligoclonal bands (OCBs) are particularly important here and are reported on in more detail in Chap. 5.

2.2.6 CIS: The Clinically Isolated Syndrome

What would happen if a patient had MS-typical symptoms and the MRI also showed MS-typical lesions in several places (dissemination in space fulfilled), but the necessary criterion of dissemination in time was missing? In this case, one speaks of a "clinically isolated syndrome" (CIS) and not yet of MS!

Since the criterion of dissemination in time is (still) missing in CIS, a prompt MRI follow-up is recommended (usually after 3 or 4 months) in order to recognise a possibly increasing activity of the disease at an early stage. If new lesions then appear in the follow-up MRI, the proof of the multiple time (dissemination in time) is provided and the diagnosis changes from CIS to MS.

MRI thus enables a rapid diagnosis and makes early treatment possible in the first place.

2.2.7   Changed Diagnostic Criteria Since 2017

With increasing knowledge about the disease, not only do the therapies change, but also some diagnostic criteria. For example, since 2017, there have been changed diagnostic criteria, the so-called "revised McDonald criteria", in which the cerebrospinal fluid examination has become significantly more important. What is new is that the detection of a certain marker in the cerebrospinal fluid, the so-called oligoclonal bands (OCBs), can replace the criterion of dissemination in time (DIT). According to these new criteria, the diagnosis of MS can thus also be made without the dissemination of space if positive OCBs can be detected in the cerebrospinal fluid.

> This has significantly increased the importance of cerebrospinal fluid examination for early diagnosis (Chap. 5).

As you can see, clear criteria are very important for diagnosing MS. Repeated changes in these guidelines over the years have led to the fact that the MS diagnosis can now be made increasingly earlier, which in turn is the basis for an early start of therapy.

> With a chronic disease like MS, which usually requires a long treatment, it is important to make the right diagnosis and to do so as early as possible!

The first two chapters, "What Is MS?" and "Do I Really Have MS?", have now given you an overview of the disease and the necessary examination methods.

In the following three chapters, we will now go into more depth, first with a "trip into our immune system" (Chap. 3). Here, you will learn more about the autoimmune process with the "players" involved. Then, in the detailed MRI chapter, we look at why the MRI is so important. Using many MRI images, I show and explain the typical MS changes (Chap. 4). And for those who want to know in more detail what cerebrospinal fluid is all about, this is followed by the chapter "The Most Important Things About Cerebrospinal Fluid" (Chap. 5).

3

A Trip into Our Immune System

3.1 The Players in Our Immune System: Lymphocytes, Antibodies and Others.

So that we understand the autoimmune process that causes MS, let us take a quick trip into our immune system. As many very different cells are involved in the disease process of MS, let us first take a closer look at the essential "players" (Fig. 3.1). These are:

– Macrophages
– Dendritic cells (DCs)
– B lymphocytes
– Plasma cells with antibodies
– Naive (i.e. not yet activated) T lymphocytes (TN)
– Regulatory T lymphocytes (T-reg)
– Activated T lymphocytes (Th1 and Th17)

Before we take a closer look at the tasks of the individual players, let us first have a look at where the cells actually come from.

A. Friedrich, *The Multiple Sclerosis Companion*, https://doi.org/10.1007/978-3-662-67540-3_3

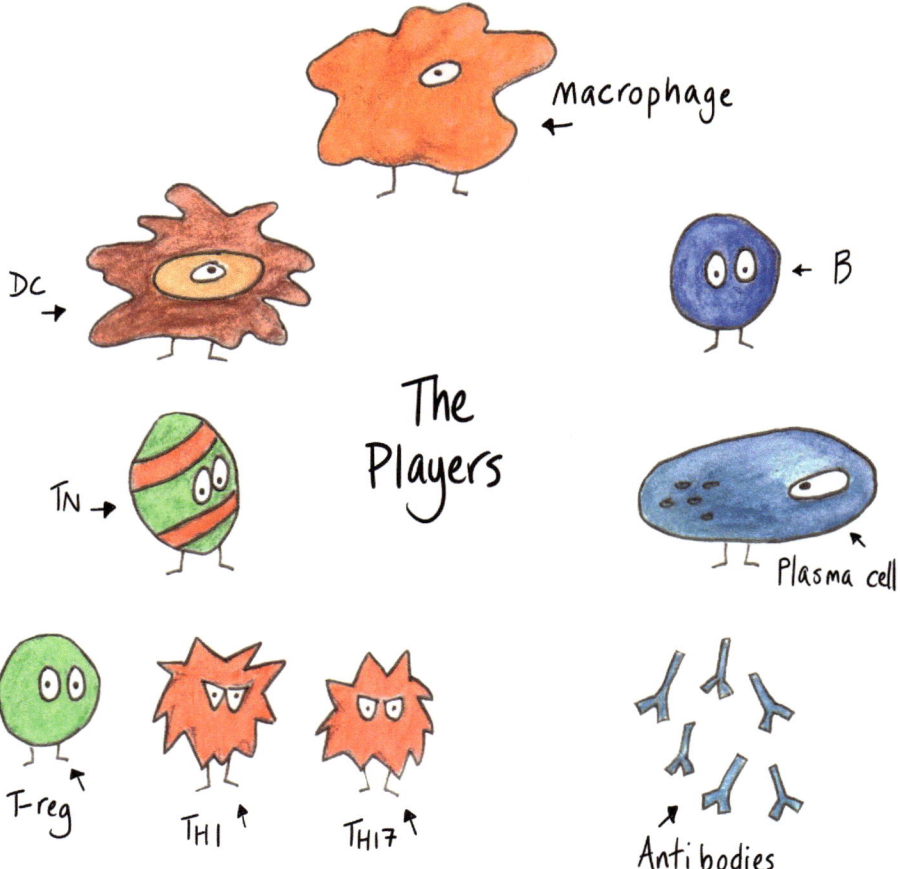

Fig. 3.1 The players of the immune system in MS

3.1.1 The Stem Cell in the Bone Marrow: The "Mother" of the Immune System

All cells develop from a common stem cell. This "mother" of the immune system is located in the bone marrow, which is a sponge-like tissue within the large bones of our body. Bone marrow, and thus the birthplace of the "mother cell", is found primarily in the vertebrae, the long bones of the arms and legs, the hip bones, the shoulder blades, the ribs and also the sternum and the bones of the skull. Two cell branches initially develop from this stem cell: the lymphoid and the myeloid precursor cell (Fig. 3.2).

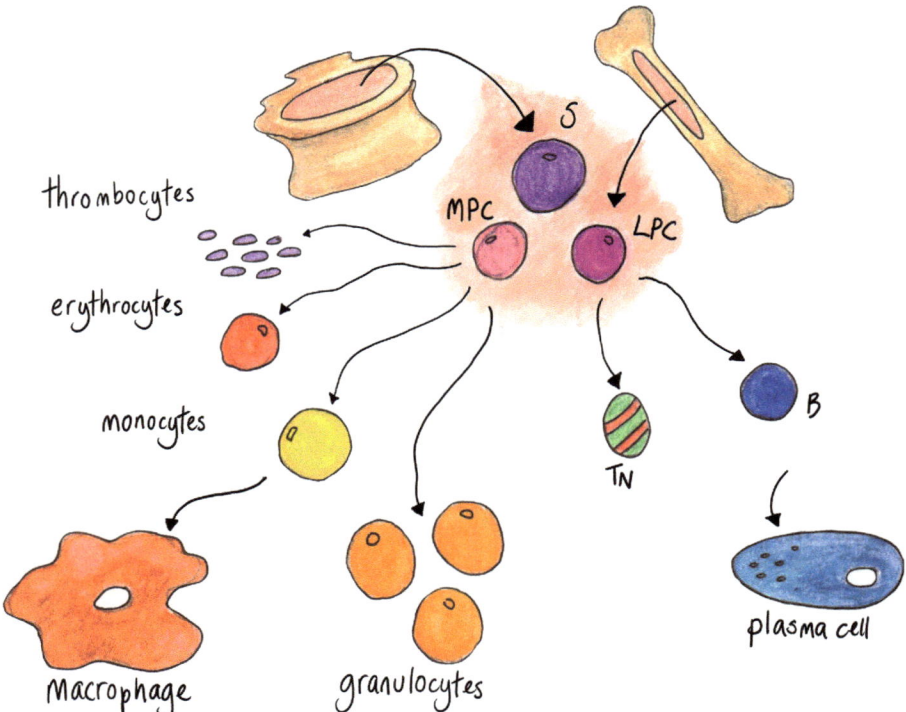

Fig. 3.2 Bone marrow with stem cell (SC), lymphoid progenitor cell (LPC) and myeloid progenitor cell (MPC)

3.1.2 The Lymphoid and the Myeloid Progenitor Cell

The lymphoid progenitor cell produces the lymphocytes, subdivided into T lymphocytes and B lymphocytes. The myeloid progenitor cell produces the granulocytes and the monocytes. In addition, the blood platelets (thrombocytes), which are responsible for blood clotting, and the red blood cells (erythrocytes), which transport oxygen in the blood, also develop from the myeloid progenitor cell. We can ignore platelets and erythrocytes from now on in this book, as they are not essential for the immune process of MS.

3.1.3 The White Blood Cells: "The Police" in the Blood

Granulocytes, monocytes and also lymphocytes belong to the group of so-called white blood cells, also called **leukocytes** in medical jargon.

As the "police in the blood", leukocytes protect our body because they serve to ward off dangers such as bacterial or viral infections. They are also important players in the autoimmune process of MS.

For example, in the case of a febrile infection, your doctor will determine a so-called "differential blood count". This examines which cells occur in the blood and how often. In the differential blood count, the leukocytes are broken down into granulocytes, monocytes and lymphocytes, i.e. "differentiated". The normal distribution of these cells in the blood looks like this:

– Granulocytes 55–75%
– Monocytes 2–6%
– Lymphocytes 25–40%

However, the values can change if inflammation is present.

3.1.4   The Innate Immune System: Granulocytes, Monocytes and Macrophages

The **granulocytes** make up the largest group of white blood cells (55–75%). They belong to the so-called innate immune system and ward off infections caused by bacteria, viruses, fungi or parasites. The **monocytes**, which also belong to this system (2–6%), can migrate from the blood into the tissue and transform into **macrophages ("big eaters").** Monocytes and macrophages are cells that recognise and destroy foreign structures by absorbing ("eating up") them. In addition to pathogens, they also eliminate dead cells and foreign bodies and are thus a kind of "rubbish disposal" of the immune system.

The innate immune system does not work specifically, which means that the reaction to intruders or foreign bodies is not targeted, i.e. the enemy is not known by name; it is only roughly recognised as "bad for the body", and an attempt is made to render it harmless—and as quickly as possible. The reaction is therefore "unspecific".

> The innate immune system serves to react quickly and non-specifically to an intruder that is recognised by the system as foreign to the body.

3.1.5   The Acquired Immune System: T and B Lymphocytes

Besides the innate immune system, there is the acquired immune system.

> The acquired immune system works much more purposefully than the innate immune system and is capable of learning.

This part of the immune system includes the **lymphocytes**. With 25–40% of all white blood cells, the lymphocytes also represent a large group of blood cells and are divided into **T** and **B lymphocytes**. As part of the acquired immune defence, they have the task of targeted, specific defence against an intruder or enemy, which they recognise and destroy. However, the prerequisite for such a targeted defence is that a lymphocyte also recognises an enemy as such, i.e. it must be able to distinguish between "endogenous" and "exogenous". But how can our immune system distinguish between endogenous and exogenous? This "learning process" takes place during lymphocyte maturation.

3.1.6   Friend or Foe: The Maturation Process of T Lymphocytes and Immunological Imprinting

The maturation process of the T lymphocytes begins before birth in the thymus gland. The thymus is an organ located in the thorax directly behind the upper third of the breastbone. This gland begins its work early, even before birth, and then continues to grow after birth, only to shrink again after puberty, until in old age it consists only of fat and connective tissue. So, the thymus is mainly active in childhood and adolescence, and that is where the "learning process" takes place, as far as "endogenous" and "exogenous" are concerned. The thymus is therefore a kind of school for the T lymphocytes. There, they get their immunological imprint, i.e. they learn to distinguish surface structures of their own body cells from surface structures foreign to the body.

But how is the child's body supposed to know what is foreign to the body if it has not yet encountered something "foreign" at birth and in its early years? How is it supposed to know which viruses or bacteria it will encounter in the course of its life? Since the child does **not** know what they will encounter later in life and which "enemies" must be fought, they cannot prepare themselves for the specific enemy. The immunological imprinting must therefore take place the other way round.

> The lymphocytes have to learn what is endogenous, what is "self", so that they later recognise the enemy because it is "not self", i.e. "not endogenous".

During the maturation process of the lymphocytes in the "thymus school", the T lymphocytes form certain T-cell receptors. These newly formed

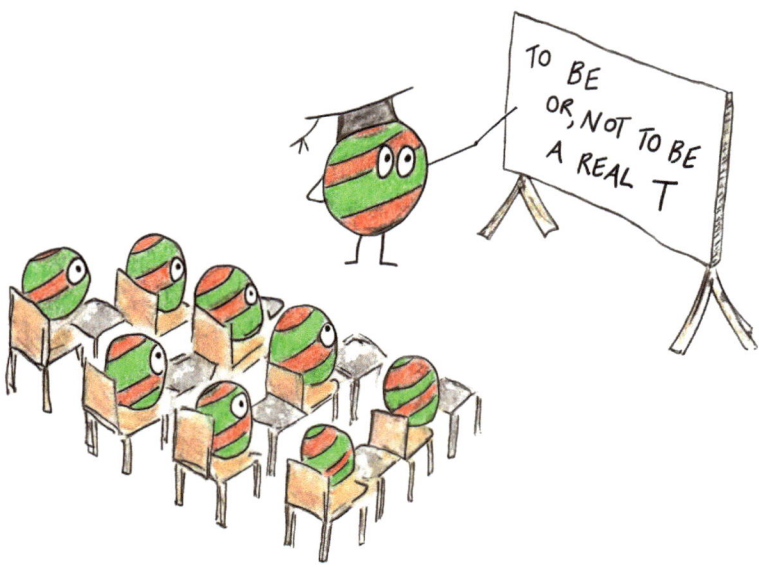

Fig. 3.3 The maturation process of T lymphocytes in the "thymus school"

receptors are subsequently tested in the thymus for their ability to recognise "endogenous". This means that in the thymus only those T cells that have formed T-cell receptors that do **not** react with surface structures of the body's own cells are allowed to leave the school successfully. Only the lymphocytes that are able to recognise "self" receive a growth signal and are allowed to "leave school", and the others die. A very strict selection is carried out here (Fig. 3.3).

These strict selection criteria mean that only about 5% of the T lymphocytes formed are allowed to successfully leave the thymus school. From there, they are then sent into the bloodstream. The others die and do not enter the blood.

This learning of so-called "self-tolerance" is extremely important so that the immune cells do not attack their own body later on, which could lead to autoimmune diseases.

For a long time, multiple sclerosis was thought to be a pure T-cell disease. Since we now know that B cells also play an important role in the disease process with myelin destruction, we are going to have a closer look at B lymphocytes.

3.1.7 The B Lymphocytes and the Perfect Defence

Unlike T lymphocytes, B cells grow in the bone marrow and undergo their maturation process there. In the course of this process, they also form special surface receptors, the B-cell receptors. Similar to T-cell maturation in the thymus, B cells also learn to recognise "the body's own" during their maturation process in the bone marrow. B cells that react to the body's own surface structures during their maturation also die.

As there is an innate and an acquired immune system, both with the same goal, it makes sense that they communicate with each other.

> For it is only through the excellent cooperation of the innate, fast but non-specific working immune system with the acquired, slower but more specific working immune system that a perfect defence is created.

What exactly this perfect defence looks like and how "the players" work together in it, we will see in the following.

3.1.8 The Phagocytes: "Big Eaters"

The body's first defence against an infection begins by activating the innate immune system. Due to the large phagocytes, such as granulocytes, monocytes and macrophages, this defence initially consists mainly of "eating". Phagocytes work by taking on the invader recognised as foreign inside the cell and breaking it down into individual parts (proteins). Pieces of these individual parts are then presented to the lymphocytes on the surface of the phagocyte as a so-called "antigen". This is comparable to putting up a mugshot so that the other immune cells can more quickly recognise which "baddie" is up to mischief and can therefore be eliminated. This is why these large cells are also called antigen-presenting cells (APCs) (Fig. 3.4).

In addition to granulocytes, monocytes and macrophages, another cell type plays an important role: the dendritic cell (DC) which also belongs to the antigen-presenting cells (APCs). The dendritic cells develop from monocytes or also from precursor cells of the B and T cells. Their main task is also the recognition of an intruder and the antigen presentation of foreign cell

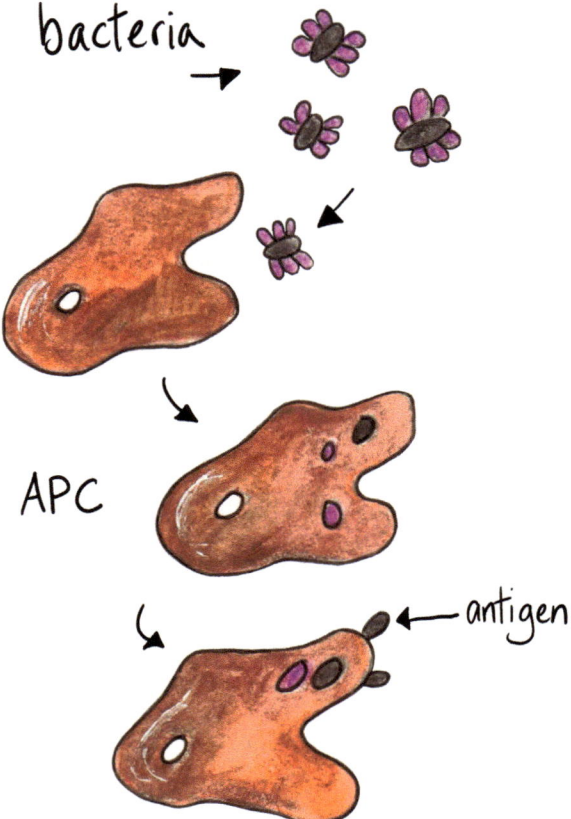

Fig. 3.4 Large phagocyte functions as an antigen-presenting cell (APC) and presents the antigen on its cell surface

structures on their cell surface. Through the presentation, the cells of the innate immune system show, as already described above: "Here is a piece of enemy, please fight!". In the illustration (Fig. 3.4), a bacterium was sketched as an example of an intruder. The presentation of the bacterial antigen on the cell surface of the APC cell activates the innate immune system, which mainly consists of T and B lymphocytes.

The antigen-presenting cells are thus the link between the innate and the acquired immune system.

3.1.9 T Lymphocyte Activation: Here We Go!

Contact between presented antigen on the surface of the large APC cell and a T lymphocyte starts T lymphocyte activation.

A so-called "naive" T lymphocyte (TN)—naive because it has not yet been activated by an antigen—binds with its T-cell receptor to the antigen presented. This activation causes the release of messenger substances, so-called cytokines, which then leads to the proliferation of the naive T lymphocytes ("expansion"). Subsequently, the T cells develop further into inflammation-firing Th1 and Th17 lymphocytes ("differentiation"), which are then able to act specifically and purposefully against the "invader" and destroy it (Fig. 3.5).

3.1.10 The Counterparts: The Regulatory T Lymphocytes

While the Th1 and Th17 lymphocytes fire up the inflammatory process, there are also T lymphocytes that down-regulate this fuelling of the inflammation so that the attack does not overshoot the target and cause more harm than good. These T lymphocytes are called regulatory T cells or T-reg for short. They are thus a kind of "brake" on the inflammatory process so that it does not get out of control (Fig. 3.6).

3.1.11 B Lymphocyte Activation, Plasma Cells and Custom-Made Antibodies

Not only the cells themselves, but also their messenger substances participate in the immune process. There are messenger substances (such as interleukin-17 = IL-17) that drive the inflammatory process, while there are also inhibitory messengers (such as interleukin-10 = IL-10).

But it is not only the T lymphocytes and messengers shown above that react when an enemy enters the body; the B lymphocytes also take up their work and join in the defence. When B lymphocytes are activated by foreign antigens from an intruder via their B-cell receptor, B lymphocyte activation begins.

> The B lymphocytes then migrate as activated B cells to the lymphatic organs, such as lymph nodes and spleen, where they multiply rapidly and subsequently transform into the so-called plasma cells. Plasma cells are the production site for antibodies.

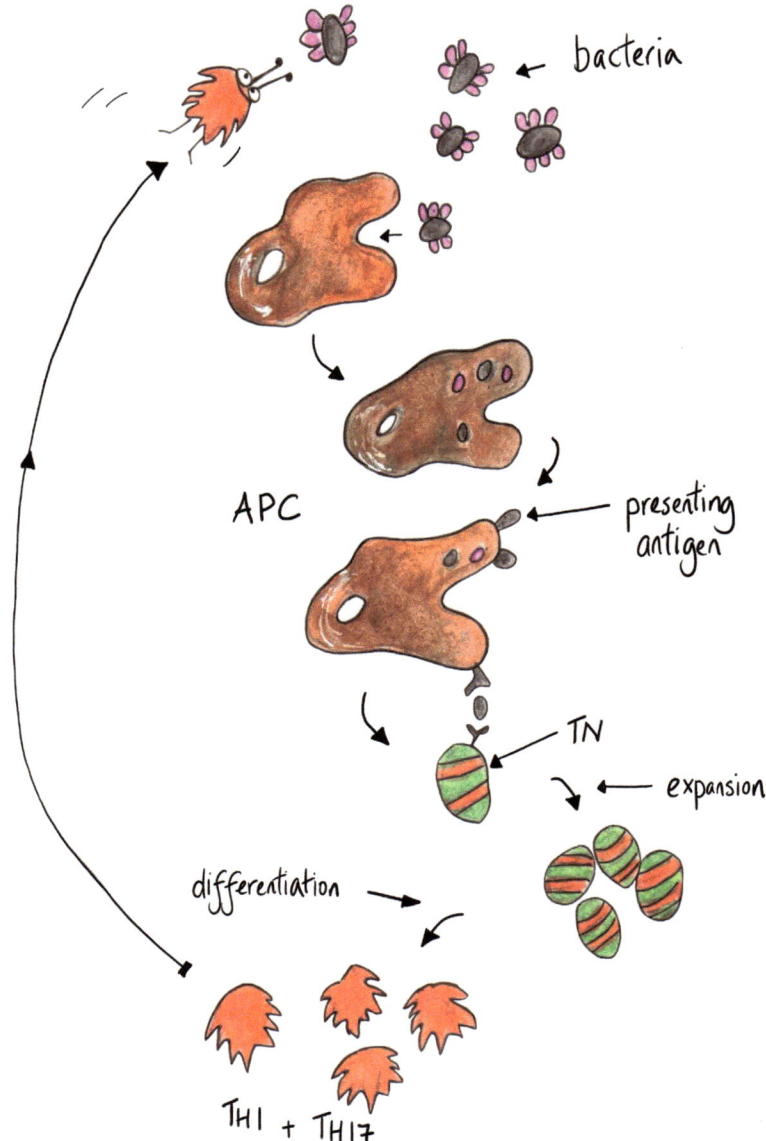

Fig. 3.5 Antigen presentation by APC cell and T lymphocyte activation

In the case of an inflammatory process, the plasma cells begin their production and form a large amount of uniform antibodies. Antibodies are small proteins, also called immunoglobulins, which are **specifically** produced against the antigen of the intruder. These antibodies are kind of "custom-made", so to speak, and fit exactly to the foreign protein of the invader by

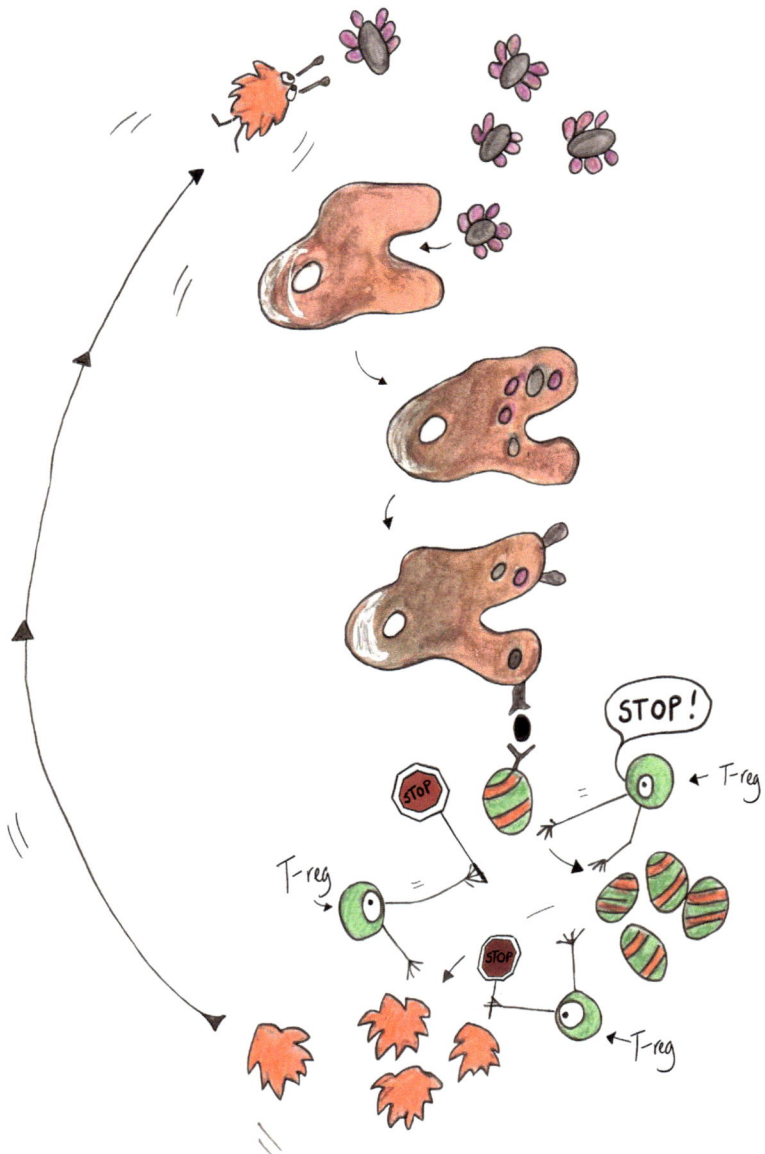

Fig. 3.6 T-reg lymphocytes at work slowing down the inflammatory process

which the B cell was initially activated via its B-cell receptor, similar to a key that only fits into a certain lock. Thus, the intruder is attacked and destroyed by the "custom-made" antibodies that are specifically and only directed against it (Fig. 3.7).

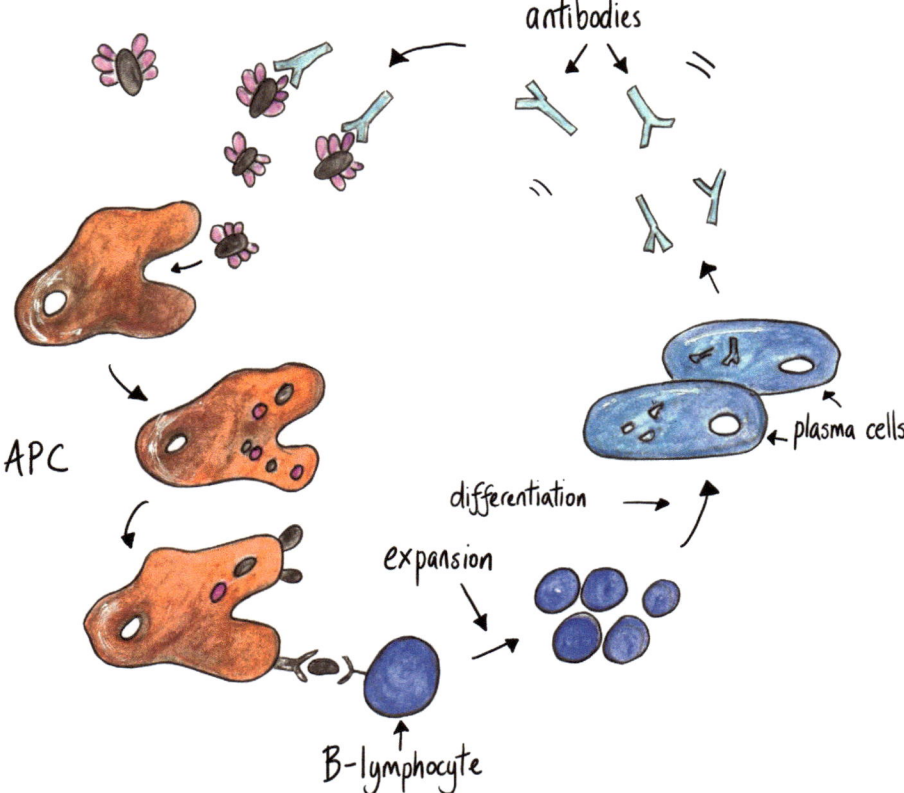

Fig. 3.7 B lymphocyte activation, plasma cell formation and antibody production

3.1.12   Reminder: The Memory Cell

In addition to this infection defence mechanism, the immune system has also come up with a kind of "reminder", a reminder function in case the same intruder should visit the body again later. Because parallel to the formation of the plasma cell, there is also the formation of a so-called memory cell. The memory cells "remember" if a similar enemy (same antigen) should later attack the body. In this case, the memory cells are activated directly, so that a specific defence against infection with antibody production can occur much more quickly in the case of a repeated infection. Often, the symptoms of the disease are milder or even completely absent.

> The immune system is therefore a very finely tuned system consisting of many components of large and small cells, messenger substances, antibodies and additional memory function.

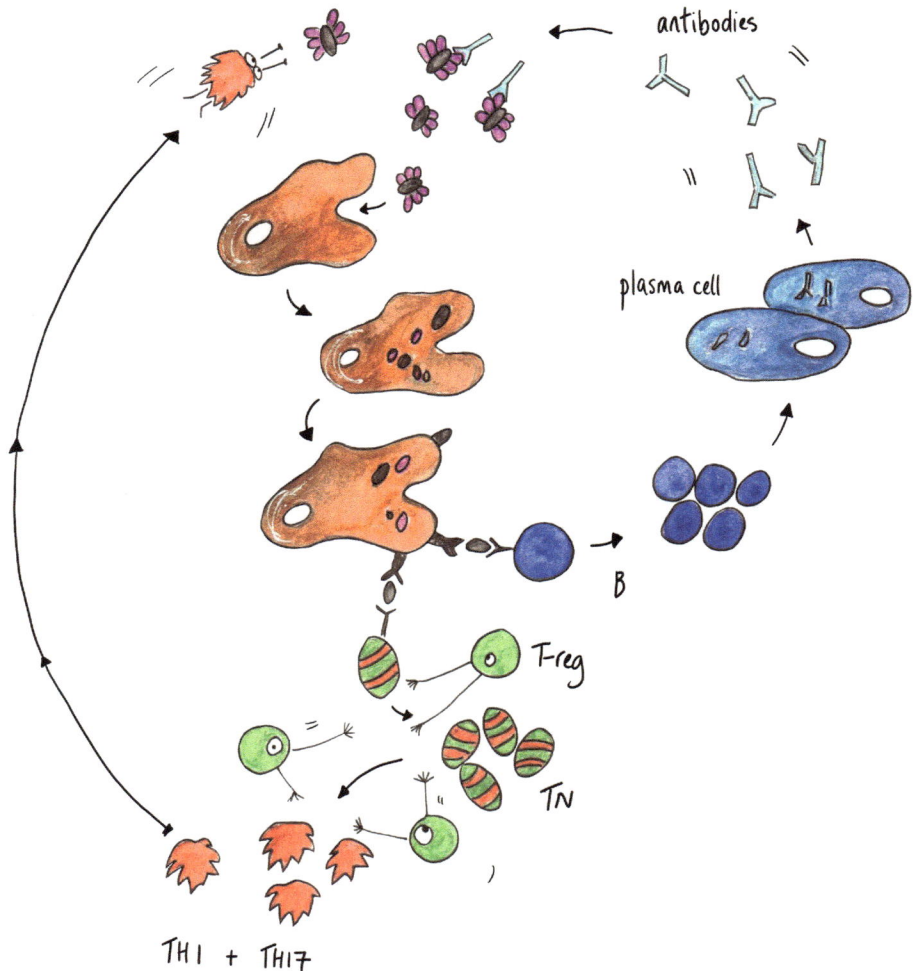

Fig. 3.8 Innate and acquired immune systems work together in defence against infection

The large phagocytes of the innate immune system, such as granulocytes, monocytes, macrophages and dendritic cells, work together with the acquired immune system of T and B lymphocytes, plasma cells and antibodies until the enemy is killed. In this way, the body is efficiently protected from invaders (Fig. 3.8).

Now that you have become acquainted with the individual players of the immune system and their tasks in the defence against infections, in the following section, we will look at how all this relates to MS.

3.2 The Inflammatory Attack Against the Nervous System

First of all, what is described above is the ideal scenario of how the immune system should function. Unfortunately, the teaching in the immune school does not always seem to go perfectly, because otherwise there would be no autoimmune diseases, i.e. diseases in which the body turns its defences against itself.

In MS, the same inflammatory process we have already learned about, which serves to protect the body from invaders, now turns against the body's own structures—in this case against the myelin. Myelin, i.e. the insulating coating of the nerve cells (Chap. 1), is attacked by the body's own immune system. What is going on? Did the T lymphocytes learn badly in their thymus school? Why is the body attacking itself? If we knew this, the cause of MS could probably be treated or even cured.

A possible explanation could be the similarity of a foreign particle in the blood with myelin. In the blood, the large phagocytes would then present an antigen that resembles the myelin that looks like its twin, so to speak. This would trigger the acquired immune system with T and B lymphocytes to attack this antigen, and it would no longer be possible to distinguish easily between the body's own myelin and the truly foreign one—they would then both simply be "enemies" on the wanted list.

3.2.1 Activated T Lymphocytes Invade the Brain

So what would happen? A T lymphocyte (T-naive cell, TN) recognises the presented surface structure as foreign to the body with its T-cell receptor and binds the presented antigen to its receptor. The receptor binding activates the T-naive lymphocyte, and it multiplies in order to be able to fight the supposed invader better with a larger force (expansion). These activated T lymphocytes develop further into the inflammation-firing (pro-inflammatory) Th1 and Th17 cells (differentiation). And now it happens: The activated Th1 and Th17 lymphocytes now search the body for their target antigen and also find it—in the CNS.

The activated lymphocytes are in fact able to migrate from the blood through the blood–brain barrier (BBB) into the brain. There, arriving on the other side in the central nervous system, they meet their target, the myelin, and attack it (Fig. 3.9).

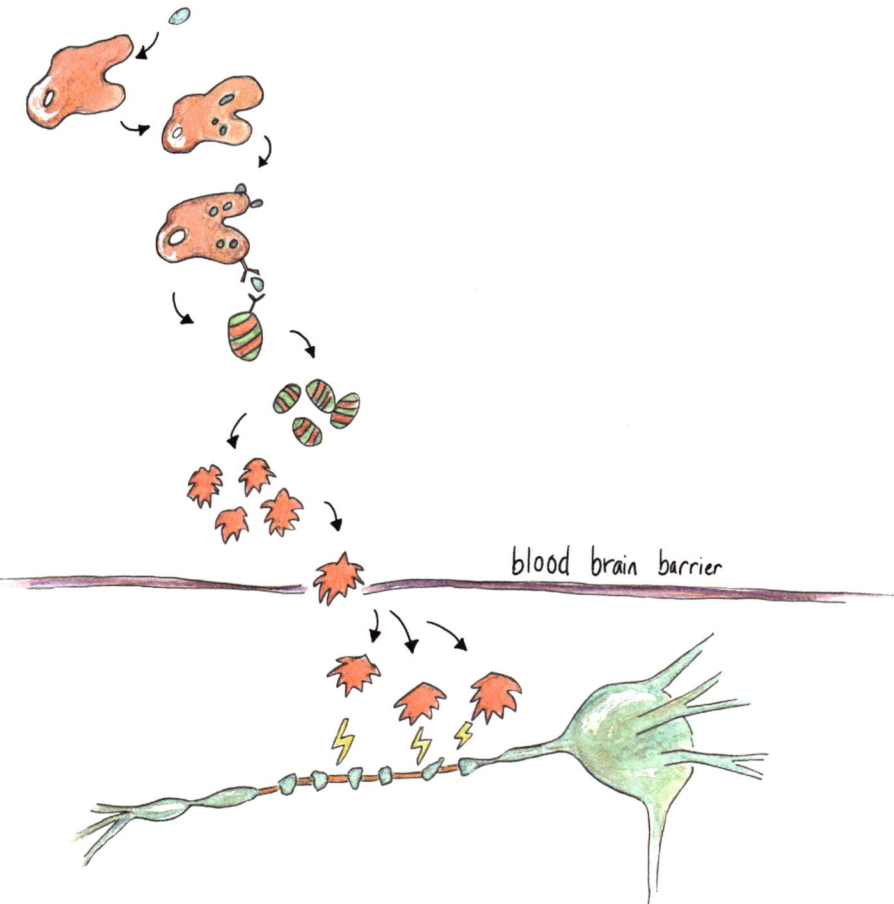

blood brain barrier

Fig. 3.9 T lymphocyte activation, passage of the blood–brain barrier and attack on the myelin

3.2.2 T Lymphocytes in Imbalance: The T-Regulatory Cells Are Weakening

This inflammation-firing process is joined by the immune system's counterparts, the regulatory T lymphocytes (T-reg). They try to counteract the inflammatory process on both sides of the blood–brain barrier in order to weaken it (Fig. 3.10).

But they do not make it.

This is because in the disease process of MS, the regulatory T cells (T-reg) are less in number, are less functional and thus have less ability to suppress the inflammatory process.

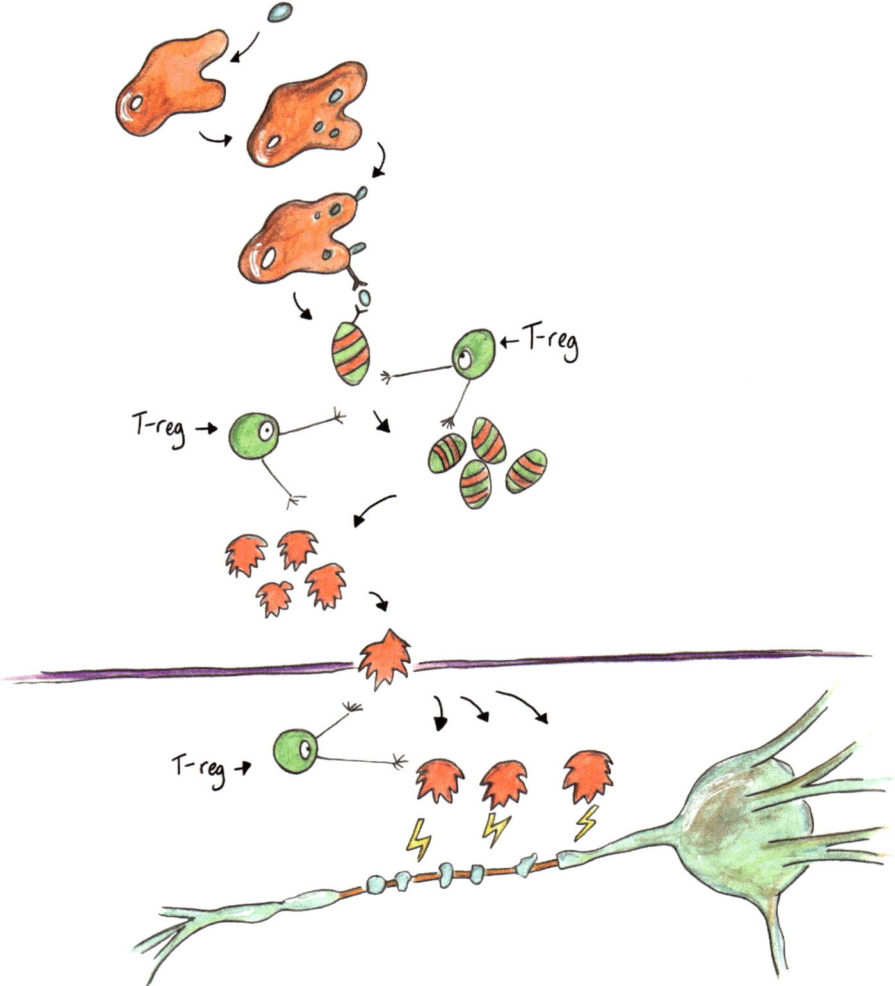

Fig. 3.10 Use of T-reg cells on this side and on the other side of the blood–brain barrier

In this way, the whole system is shifted towards "ignition firing" (Fig. 3.11).

In a sense, the inflammatory reaction brake is missing. In this way, the Th1 and Th17 lymphocytes can attack the myelin of the nerve cells in a more unchecked way.

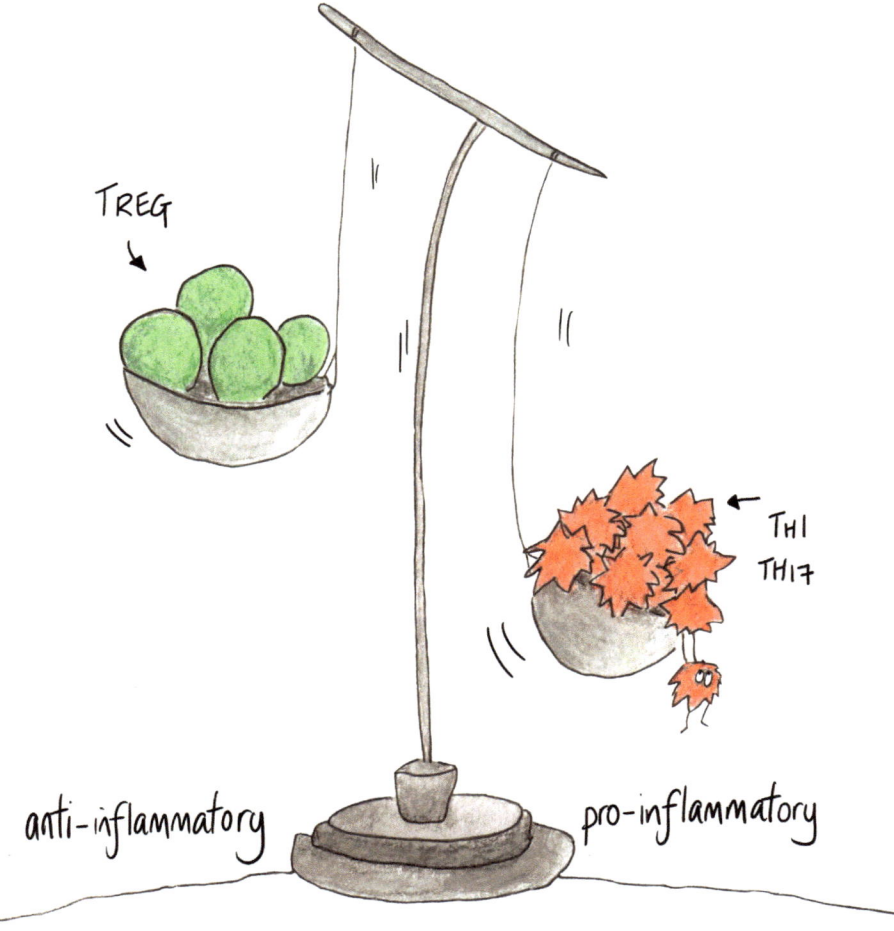

Fig. 3.11   Imbalance of T-reg and Th1/17 lymphocytes in MS

3.2.3   The Attack Against the Myelin: Common Cause with the B Lymphocytes

During this attack, the T lymphocytes are helped by other players of the immune system. In contrast to earlier thinking, MS is not a pure T-cell disease. The B lymphocytes also play a role in this disease process and for a long time were not given sufficient consideration. Not only the activated T lymphocytes, but also the activated B cells can cross the blood–brain barrier and support the inflammatory process through plasma cell formation and antibody production against the myelin.

> Th1 and Th17 T cells, together with the B cells and their plasma cells with antibodies, carry out the inflammatory attack against the nervous tissue (Fig. 3.12).

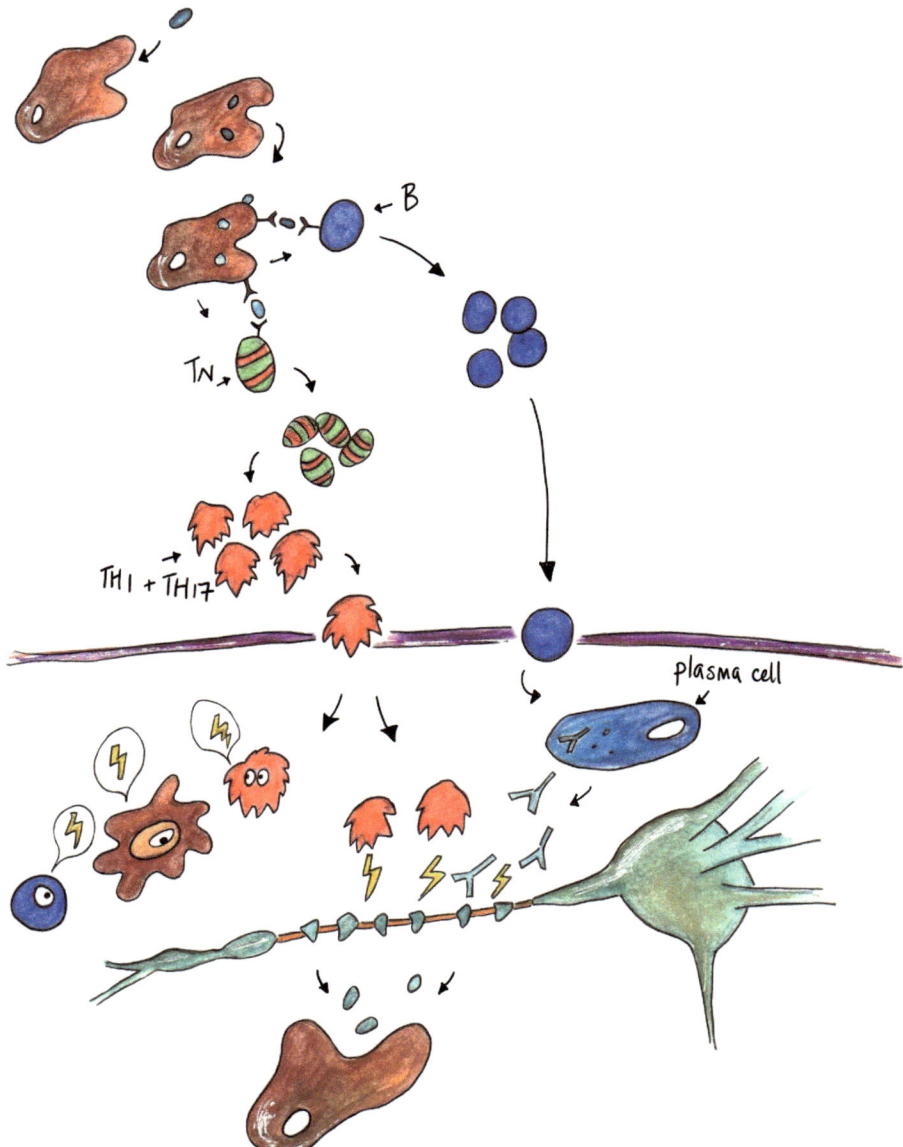

Fig. 3.12 Common attack in the CNS against the myelin of the nerve cells

The result is "cable breaks and short circuits" of the axons, so that information can no longer be passed from one nerve cell to the next. The final state is complete "cable damage", a demyelinated axon, which is soon followed by the demise of the nerve cell itself (Fig. 3.13).

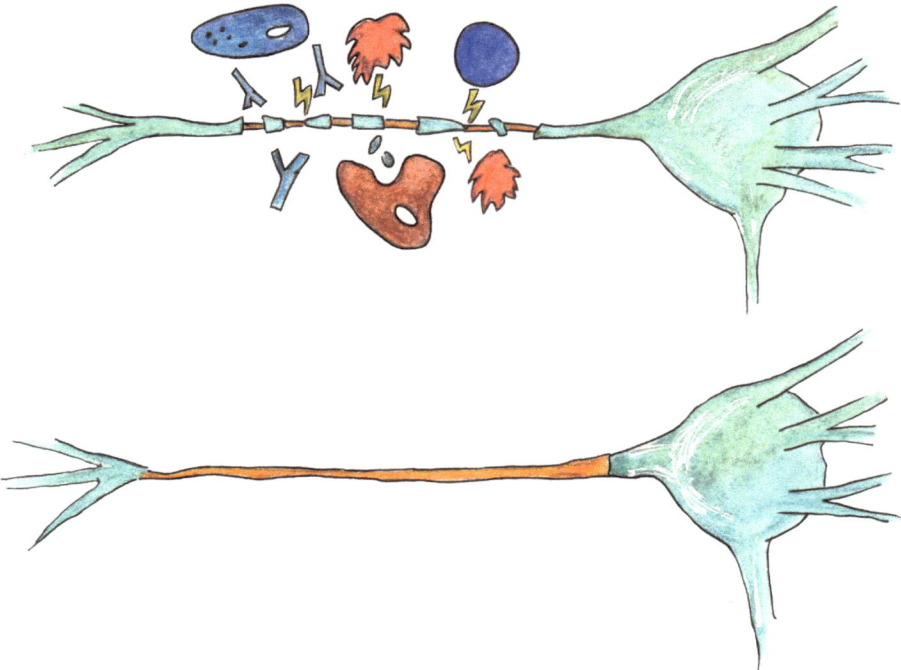

Fig. 3.13 The consequences of the inflammatory attack—demyelination with cell death

T cells trigger the inflammatory reaction in the CNS, but they are short-lived. The B cells, on the other hand, are maintained because they form memory cells that can continue to produce antibodies against the myelin. Thus, the B cells may be able to continue to maintain the inflammatory process in the CNS independently of the blood. Because of these considerations, B cells are increasingly the focus of research today.

3.2.4   B-Cell Nests: A New Discovery

There is another discovery that seems very interesting, even if it has not yet been fully clarified. So-called B-cell nests have been found in the central nervous system, especially in secondary progressive MS (SPMS). These are lymphatic organs that are supposed to be located lymph node-like on the meninges surrounding the brain. It is possible that these B-cell nests, which settle in the brain, are the cause of the disease taking on a life of its own with relapse-independent progression in the later course of the disease. The B-cell nests could possibly also explain the poor response to medication in the later course of secondary progressive MS (SPMS). It is likely that macrophages, dendritic cells and CNS-resident tissue macrophages (microglia) also maintain the inflammatory process once it has been initiated.

Now that this trip into our immune system has given you essential information about the disease mechanism of MS and you know which players are involved, in the next chapter, we will look at how the inflammatory process described here appears in the MRI.

4

Why MRI?

4.1 My MRI Report: *Not* a Closed Book!

Recognise this? You get your MRI report from the radiologist, try to read it at home and understand next to nothing. The report is peppered with many strange, foreign-sounding words and is really intended as information from doctor to doctor. Because the MRI plays a very important role today both for clarifying the MS diagnosis and for monitoring the therapy, I would like to take a closer look at this type of examination and the report of the findings. You will shortly see many different MS-typical MRI images, which will be explained in detail. Let us start with a classic MRI report, which you might not understand (yet), but will certainly understand by the end of this chapter:

Magnetic resonance imaging of the skull with and without contrast medium from (date).

"*For comparison, an external preliminary examination dated (date) is available. Evidence of numerous patchy, partly converging signal elevations, **cockscomb like** at **corpus callosum level**, in the **periventricular white matter** and **juxta-cortically** in the **T2 and T2-FLAIR sequence.** Suspicion of a small lesion on the right **cerebellar** side. The lesions are definable as **hypointense** lesions in the **native T1 sequence.** No evidence of **pathological contrast enhancement**. Somewhat accentuated inner and outer CSF spaces. As far as can be compared with the previous images, no significant change in findings compared to the previous findings*".

A. Friedrich, *The Multiple Sclerosis Companion*, https://doi.org/10.1007/978-3-662-67540-3_4

As you can see, without a certain basic knowledge of the vocabulary, such findings cannot be understood. To change that, let us have a closer look at these basics on the next few pages and the following topics:

– Anatomical terms you should know.
– Where MS occurs.
– How the MRI works.
– How the MRI is read: The image contrasts.
– Why the contrast agent is important.
– What "black holes", "footprints" and brain atrophy mean.
– When an MRI is necessary.
– Examples of MS-typical MRI images.

With this information, it will then be easy for you to better understand an MRI report in the future and to recognise the decisive information on the MRI images.

4.2   Anatomical Terms You Should Know

MRI stands for magnetic resonance imaging and is also called nuclear spin tomography. Tomography is derived from the Greek word for "section", and that is exactly what happens with an MRI: sectional images of the human body are created at any level, which, when put together, give a more complete overall impression. The advantage is that you can look at the corresponding anatomical structures in detail from different perspectives and thus better judge normal or pathologically changed regions.

> The MRI generates sectional images of the human body in any plane.

In order for orientation to be successful, these sectional planes must be defined. Three standardised axes are used for imaging the brain and spinal cord, which you can find in the following figure.

These three standardised sectional planes (Fig. 4.1) are named as follows

• The **axial plane** (shown in blue) or also called the transverse plane

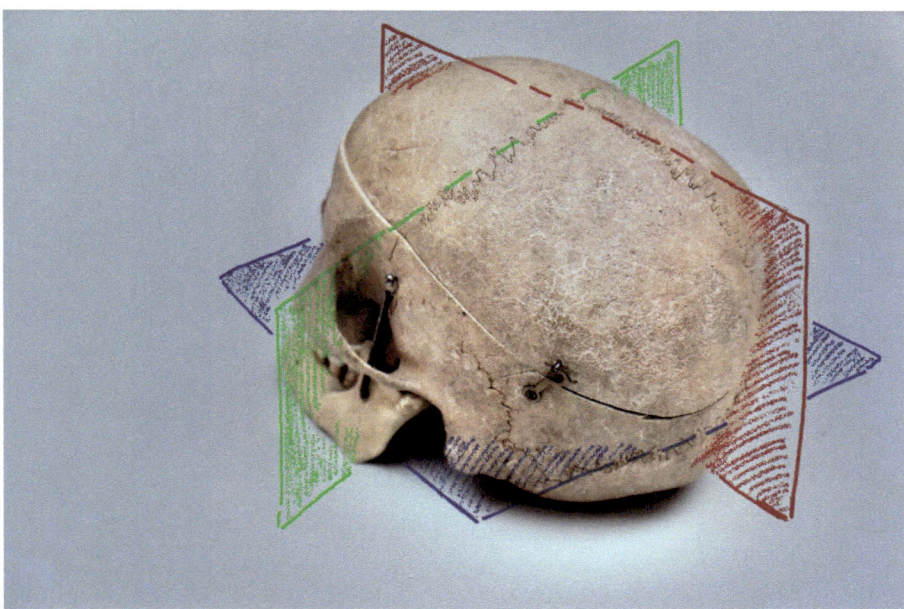

Fig. 4.1 The three sectional planes: axial (blue), sagittal (red) and coronal (green)

- The **sagittal plane** (red) named after the cranial bone suture "sutura *sagittalis*"
- The **coronal plane** (green), also called the frontal plane named after the "sutura *coronalis*"

For the MS examination, the axial and sagittal, i.e. lateral, sectional planes are particularly important. You can see below what the individual sectional planes look like in the MRI and what can be seen particularly well and on which plane.

4.2.1 The Brain in Slices: The Axial Sectional Plane in MRI

Let us start with the axial sectional plane and look at the figure below for a better understanding. The best way to think of the axial sectional plane is as if you were slicing a bread roll lengthwise. Each slice is looked at, and you can easily imagine that the slice thickness is very important here. In a similar way, you can look at each layer of the brain in the MRI, and the thinner the individual slices, the more information you get. In the axial plane, the upper edge of the image shows the frontal area, and the lower edge shows the back of the

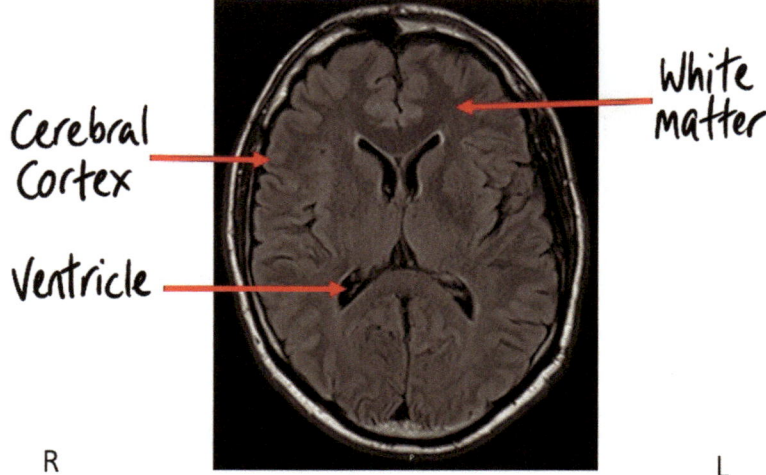

Fig. 4.2 Axial sectional plane

head. The right and left sides are marked with "R" and "L", but be careful: R and L appear laterally reversed in the MRI image (Fig. 4.2).

4.2.2 Cortex, White Matter and Ventricles: Where Do I Find What?

In the axial sectional plane, the cerebral **cortex** is clearly visible (Fig. 4.2). The cortex surrounds the brain like a coat and has a folded appearance. The many thousands of cell bodies of the nerve cells are located here. The cortex is folded to increase surface area. You can also see the **white matter** in the axial sectional plane—this is where the axons are located, i.e. the "connecting cables" that pass on the information to the different regions of the brain. On the very inside are the **ventricles**, which are the brain chambers that contain cerebrospinal fluid. In the ventricles, the cerebrospinal fluid is formed, and this washes around the brain and spinal cord and thus cushions the central nervous system and protects it. More about the cerebrospinal fluid follows in Chap. 5.

4.2.3 The Brain in Longitudinal Section: The Corpus Callosum and the Roof of the Cerebellum in Focus

In the sagittal plane, i.e. the lateral view of the brain, the cerebrum, the cerebellum and the brainstem, which then merges into the spinal cord, are particularly well shown. An important structure is the roof of the cerebellum,

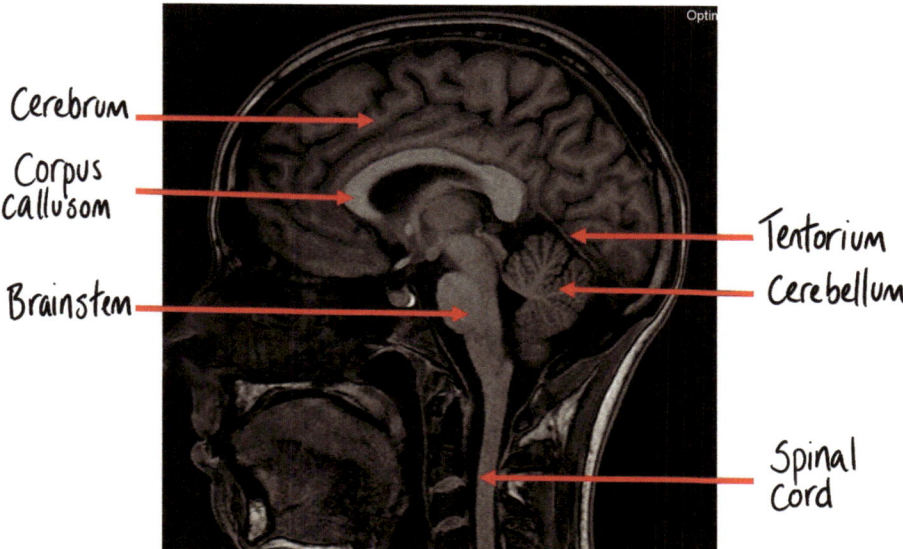

Fig. 4.3 Sagittal sectional plane

called tentorium cerebelli. The tentorium separates the cerebrum from the posterior fossa, where the cerebellum and brainstem are located. The **tentorium** is used for orientation because everything above the tentorium is called "supratentorial", and everything below the tentorium is called "infratentorial". You will find these two terms in the MRI report very often (Fig. 4.3).

An important structure in MS diagnostics is the **corpus callosum**. The nerve fibre bundles of the left and right brain hemispheres cross in the corpus callosum, thus connecting both brain hemispheres so that they can communicate with each other.

> The corpus callosum, which is particularly well displayed in the sagittal plane, is often affected by inflammatory lesions in MS and is therefore an important structure in disease detection.

4.2.4 All Good Things Come in Threes: The Coronal Plane

The third plane is the coronal plane or frontal plane. Visible here are the **cerebrum**, the **ventricles,** the **roof of the cerebellum** (tentorium) and below that the **cerebellum** (Fig. 4.4).

Now that we have gained an overview of the anatomy and the cutting planes here, we will look at where the MS-typical lesions are located in the following chapter.

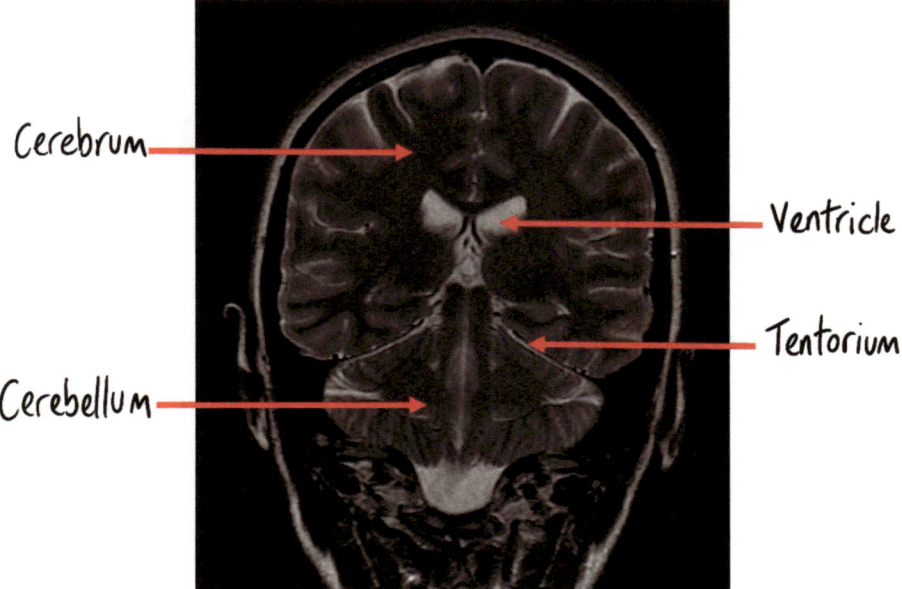

Cerebrum

Ventricle

Tentorium

Cerebellum

Fig. 4.4 Coronal sectional plane

4.3   Where MS Sits in the Body

MS lesions appear as "white spots" in most MRI images (for more on this, see Sect. 4.5). However, not every white spot is suspicious for MS. There are four typical locations in the central nervous system that are characteristic of MS lesions and should be looked at especially when there is a clinical suspicion of MS. The names for these four typical locations are also always found in the MRI report, and they are called as follows:

1. Periventricular
2. Infratentorial
3. Juxtacortical
4. Spinal

Periventricular means that the MS lesions lie **next to the** ventricles, i.e. the brain chambers, and touch them (Fig. 4.5 cf. Fig. 1, marked in red).

Infratentorial means that the MS lesions are located **below the** tentorium, i.e. in the cerebellum and/or brainstem (Fig. 4.5 Fig. 2, marked in red).

Juxtacortical means that the lesions lie in the immediate vicinity of the cortex and touch it (Fig. 4.5, Fig. 3, marked in red).

Spinal lesions are lesions in the spinal cord, i.e. lesions in the cervical or thoracic medulla (Fig. 4.6, Fig. 4 in sagittal and Fig. 5 in axial sectional plane, lesions marked in red).

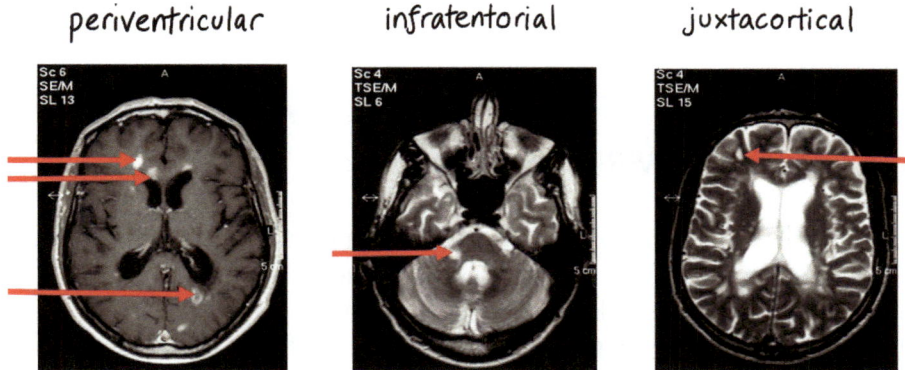

periventricular   infratentorial   juxtacortical

Fig. 4.5   Figures 1–3 MS lesions in axial sectional plane

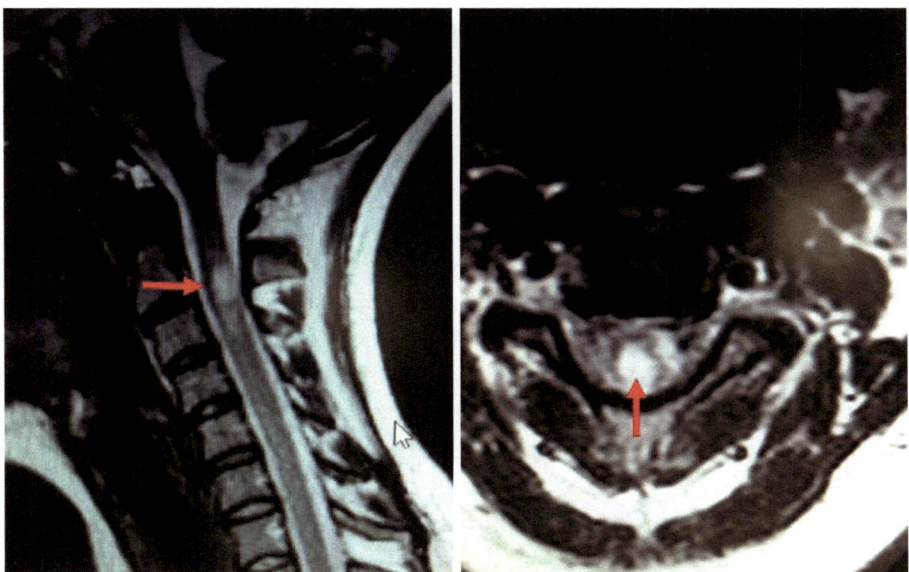

Fig. 4.6   Spinal lesions in sagittal (Fig. 4) and axial sectional plane (Fig. 5)

So, now we have looked at the typical lesion locations for MS and their names. If "white spots" are found at these locations mentioned, it could be MS.

But be careful: not every "white spot" in the brain immediately leads to an MS diagnosis!

Other criteria must be fulfilled for this, which we will return to in more detail later (Sect. 4.8).

4.4   How the MRI Works

Many of you have probably already experienced the MRI. A large, loud, tube-like device where you have to remove all metal items before the examination. Why is that? Since the MRI works with a magnetic field that is more than 60,000 times stronger than the earth's magnetic field, all metal objects are attracted to this strong magnet. Free metal objects would therefore be drawn into the MRI tube and could damage it or injure the patient. That is why metal is not allowed in the MRI room. However, the MRI does not only work with this strong magnetic field, but it uses the combination of the magnetic field and an additional high-frequency pulse (HF pulse).

4.4.1   Magnetic Field and Hydrogen Atoms

Hydrogen atoms are used for MRI imaging, which is appropriate because the human body is predominantly made up of water. An atom is a tiny structure consisting of an atomic nucleus and an atomic shell. It is invisible to the naked eye, though all matter is made of atoms. The nucleus, as the inner part of the atom, consists of a single, positively charged particle (H+) in the case of a hydrogen atom. Atomic nuclei (protons) constantly rotate around their own axis under normal conditions. This angular momentum is called nuclear spin (Fig. 4.7). This is where the other term for MRI mentioned above comes from: nuclear spin tomography. Through this intrinsic rotation, the nuclei of the hydrogen atoms generate small magnetic fields. These small magnetic fields are influenced by the large magnetic field of the MRI when the body is in the MRI.

Under natural conditions, the magnetic alignment of the many hydrogen atoms in the body is rather disordered, but this changes as soon as the body is exposed to a strong magnetic field. Due to the strong external magnetic field of the MRI, the protons in the body align themselves in an ordered manner along the main direction of the magnetic field (Fig. 4.8).

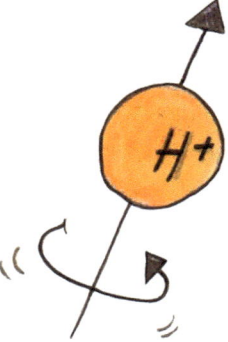

Fig. 4.7 Rotating hydrogen atomic nucleus

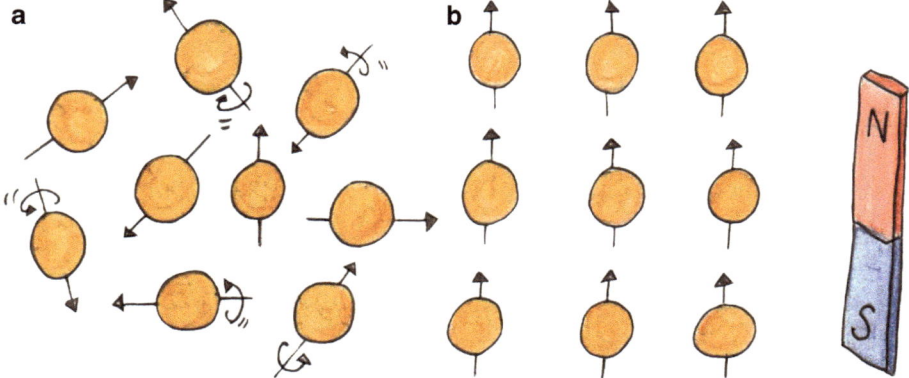

Fig. 4.8 Under natural conditions, disordered alignment of the rotating hydrogen atoms (**a**), under the influence of the magnetic field, ordered alignment (**b**)

4.4.2 High-Frequency Pulse (HF Pulse) and Hydrogen Atoms

As already mentioned, the MRI not only works with the force of the magnetic field but is also followed by a so-called high-frequency pulse (HF pulse), as a short pulse with a characteristic radio frequency.

This short impulse changes the parallel alignment of the hydrogen nuclei in the magnetic field, and the protons are additionally deflected in a different direction in a layer before they fall back into the original longitudinal direction, which is specified by the magnet. During this "falling back", the hydrogen nuclei emit signals that can be measured. Depending on the tissue-specific amount of hydrogen nuclei in the different tissues and organs of the body, these signals differ, so that different types of tissue can be distinguished from each other through the different signal behaviours. Fluid, for example, presents itself differently in the MRI than brain tissue, as Sect. 4.5 will show. To obtain an MRI image, a tissue layer must be stimulated and measured many times by the high-frequency pulse.

4.4.3 The Image Contrast: How the Different Images Are Created

The technique of MRI is very complex, and in this book, we will only be interested in two essential parameters, which are, however, very important for the image contrast of the MRI images. These two parameters are the repetition time and the echo time.

- The **repetition time** (TR = time of repetition) is the time between two successive stimulations by the high-frequency pulse in milliseconds (ms).
- The **time of echo** (TE = time of echo) is the time that passes until the signal is measured after stimulation (also called "readout time").

> By choosing different combinations of repetition time and echo time, the different image contrasts can be achieved in the MRI image.

In the next chapter, let us have a look at how different MRI images can look in different image contrasts.

4.5 How to Read the MRI: The Image Contrasts

Depending on the choice of repetition time (TR = time of repetition) and echo time (TE = time of echo), completely different-looking MRI images can be produced, because the choice of the possible combinations of TR and TE determines the image contrast. As you will see in a moment, taking into account many different image contrasts gives us more information about the brain and also about possible damage.

4.5.1   The Image Contrast T1 and T2

There are many different image contrasts. In the following, we will only be interested in the contrasts that are important for MS diagnostics. For this purpose, the T1- and T2-weighted images are important, and there are also special forms of T2 weighting for contrast enhancement. In the following, we will have a closer look at the different image contrasts. Let us start with T1 and T2 and look at the following illustration (Fig. 4.9). It shows an MRI in sagittal (top row) and axial (bottom row) sectional plane, on the left in T1

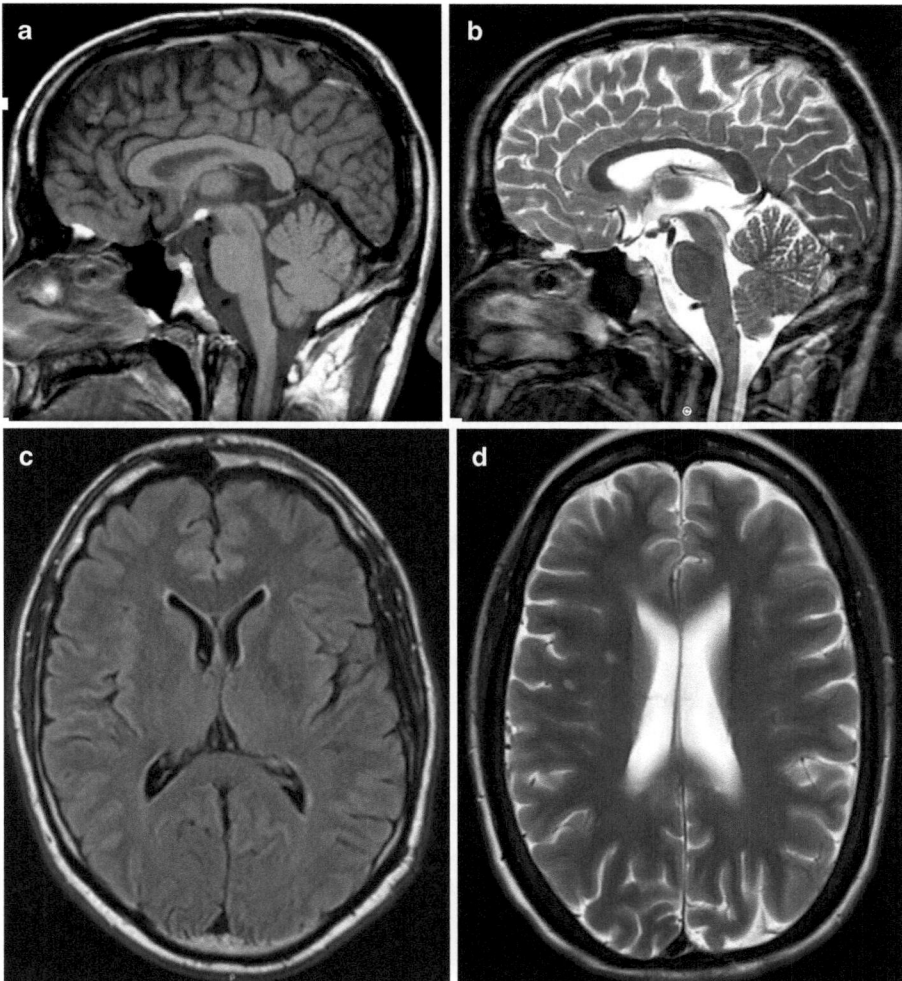

Fig. 4.9   (a–d) T1- (left) and T2- (right) weighted MRI images in sagittal (top) and axial (bottom) sectional plane

weighting and on the right in T2 weighting: two images that look quite different. The most striking difference is that the cerebrospinal fluid that fills the ventricles and washes around the brain is shown dark in T1 images, but light in T2 images.

Technically, T1-weighted images are created by a short repetition time TR (shorter than 500 ms)—i.e. high-frequency pulses that follow one another quickly—and also a short echo time TE (shorter than 20 ms)—i.e. a readout time that follows quickly and directly after the high-frequency pulse.

> In T1-weighted images, water and cerebrospinal fluid (CSF) appear dark against the brain, which is silhouetted in grey.

It is quite different in the T2-weighted MRI image, which is obtained by a long TR (longer than 2000 ms) and a late readout time TE (longer than 50 ms).

> In T2 images, water and cerebrospinal fluid appear light against the brain.

By changing the two parameters TR and TE, two very-different-looking MRI images can be produced. Not only does the cerebrospinal fluid look different in T1 and T2, but the representation of the MS lesions is also very different depending on the choice of the two parameters.

4.5.2   T1-Weighted Images: MS Lesions Can Hide

So, let us look below at what MS lesions look like in T1- and T2-weighted MRI images, starting with **T1**. In T1-weighted MRI images, MS lesions usually look like the brain tissue itself and are therefore not visible at all. Something that looks like brain tissue is known as "isointense". However, MS lesions can also look darker than the brain tissue in T1, which is then called "hypointense" (◉). (Fig. 4.10, marked with an arrow). Both are possible.

> It is important to know that MS lesions can "hide" in T1-weighted images because they can look similar to brain tissue. Therefore, the extent of MS damage cannot be assessed in T1 images.

Fig. 4.10 T1-weighted MRI with dark, hypointense MS focus in the white matter

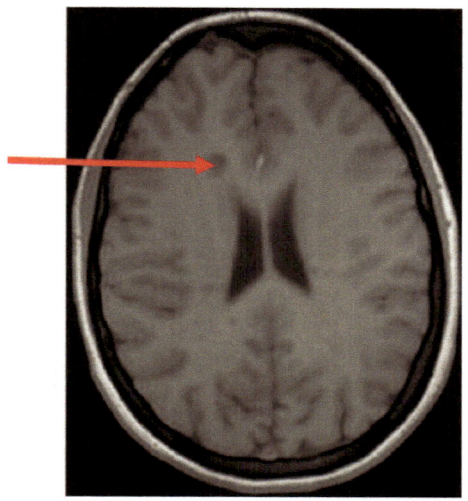

Why images are taken, in which MS lesions may not be visible at all, will only become clear to you later when we talk about the contrast medium. Before that, here is some information about the T2 image.

4.5.3   T2-Weighted Images: Here You Can See More

In T2-weighted images (Fig. 4.11), MS lesions appear lighter than brain tissue just as the cerebrospinal fluid does too, and this is called "hyperintense".

> In T2-weighted MRI images, the MS lesions always appear as the typical "white spots".

For contrast enhancement, there are special forms of T2 weighting in addition to the "normal" T2-weighted image. These are very useful in MS diagnostics. To illustrate this, we will have a closer look at these special forms in the following and also compare them with each other.

Fig. 4.11 T2-weighted MRI with many bright, hyperintense MS lesions in the white matter as typical "white spots"

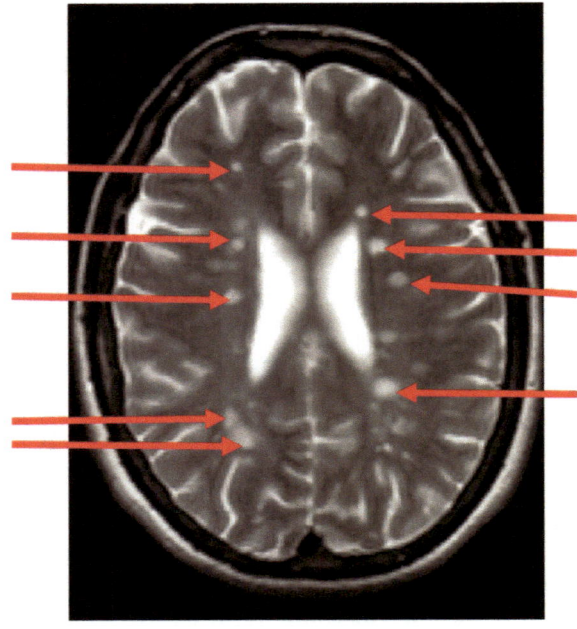

4.5.4 The T2 Special Forms: T2-FLAIR, PD and DIR Sequence

The four different T2 weightings that should be looked at in more detail are

1. T2 (long), the "normal" T2 weighting that you already know
2. T2-PD (stands for "proton density")
3. T2-FLAIR (stands for "fluid-attenuated inversion recovery")
4. DIR sequence (stands for "double-inversion recovery")

4.5.5 T2-PD: Proton Weighted

T2-PD stands for proton-weighted images. Like T2 (long), they are technically characterised by a long TR, but the TE readout time is short, which changes the image significantly compared to T2. This gives the image a somewhat "soft" appearance. The abundance of cells in the cortex leads to a stronger signal, which makes the light greyish cortex appear thicker.

> In PD images, therefore, a good distinction can be made between the cerebral cortex and the white matter.

Fig. 4.12 T2-PD sequence with many bright, hyperintense MS lesions in the white matter

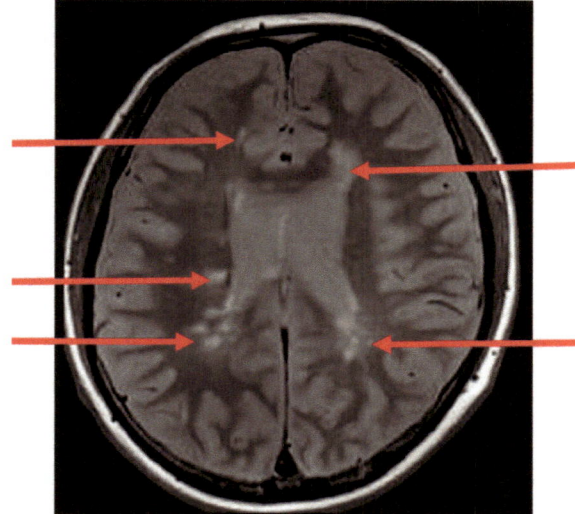

The cerebrospinal fluid in the cerebral ventricles also appears more greyish than in the T2-long image. MS lesions appear lighter (= hyperintense) in T2-PD than brain tissue (Fig. 4.12).

4.5.6 T2-FLAIR: For a Good Overview

With the T2-FLAIR sequence (fluid-attenuated inversion recovery), the signal of the free fluids (CSF) is suppressed by an additional preliminary impulse and is therefore black. As a result, the cerebrospinal fluid, which would otherwise appear light in T2-long, appears dark in T2-FLAIR.

MS lesions are also light in the T2-FLAIR sequence but are better distinguishable from the darker CSF than in T2-long. Particularly small lesions near the ventricles are more visible due to the adjacent dark CSF (Fig. 4.13).

> In the T2-FLAIR, the MS lesions stand out most against the dark CSF, so the T2-FLAIR image is often used for the initial overview.

4.5.7 The DIR Sequence: Shows Lesions in the Cerebral Cortex

In the DIR sequence (double-inversion recovery), technically not only the CSF signal is suppressed (as with T2-FLAIR), but also that of the white matter. This means that the white matter, like the CSF, is now displayed as dark.

Fig. 4.13 T2-FLAIR MRI with many bright, hyperintense MS lesions adjacent to the ventricles (periventricular)

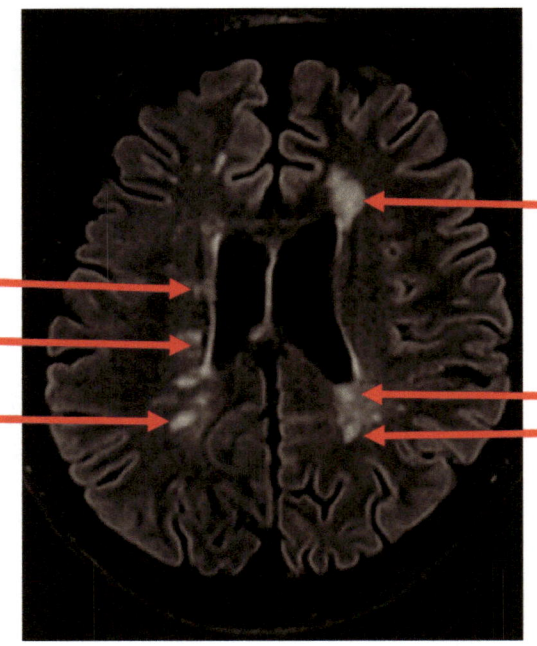

With the DIR sequence, lesions particularly close to the cortex ("juxtacortical" lesions) or lesions within the cortex ("intracortical lesions") can be made visible (Fig. 4.14).

With the older MRI methods, juxtacortical and intracortical lesions, i.e. lesions within the cerebral cortex, could not be depicted at all. Therefore, it was wrongly assumed that multiple sclerosis does not affect the cerebral cortex. This idea has since changed due to improved technical possibilities such as the DIR sequence, and it could be shown that cortical lesions can even often be present in the early stages of MS.

Now that we have got to know the T2-weighted images with their special forms PD, FLAIR and DIR, let us look at them again in direct comparison with each other. You will see that more information can be obtained when all sequences are taken into account (Fig. 4.15).

4.5.8 In a Nutshell

In summary, we can state that by changing the repetition time (TR) and the echo time (TE), different image contrasts are achieved. MS lesions are lighter than the surrounding brain tissue in **all** T2-weighted MRI images

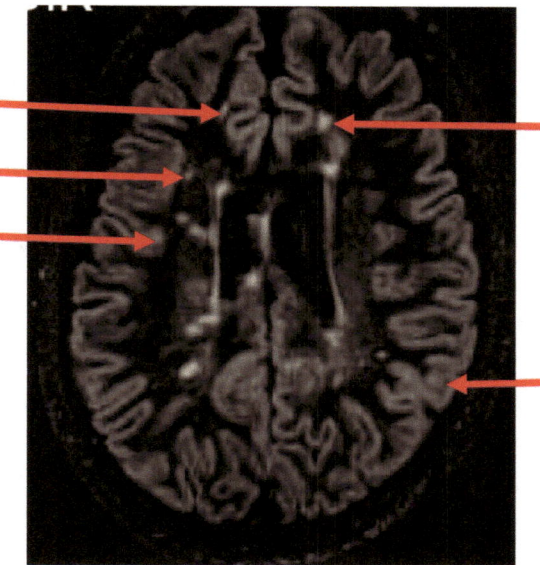

Fig. 4.14 DIR sequence: bright hyperintense MS lesions close to the cortex (juxtacortical) and within the cortex (intracortical) arrow-marked

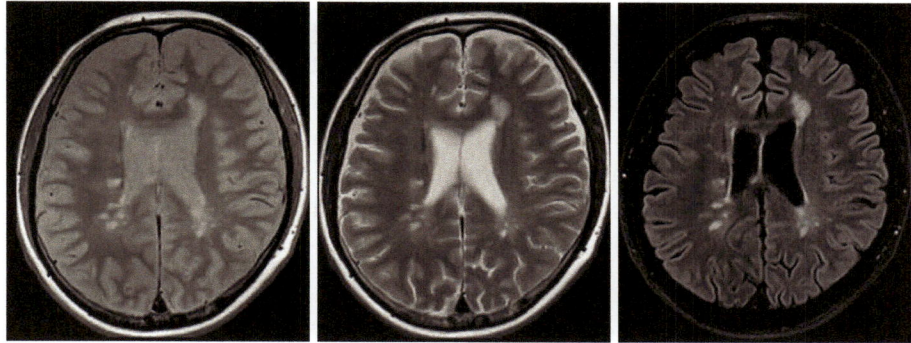

Fig. 4.15 Comparison: T2-PD, T2 (long), T2-FLAIR

(hyperintense). In T1-weighted images, on the other hand, MS lesions are often not visible at all because they look exactly like the brain tissue itself (isointense) or they are darker than brain tissue, which is then called hypointense.

> Taking into account as many different MRI image contrasts as possible gives us the opportunity to better and more completely assess the extent of MS damage.

4.6   Why the Contrast Medium Is Important

Why is the additional administration of contrast medium (or contrast agent) in an MRI so important in MS diagnostics? Apparently, a lot can be depicted even without it. In this chapter, we will look at when and why contrast medium may or may not be necessary. Today, well-tolerated contrast agents containing gadolinium are used as contrast agents.

4.6.1   The MRI Procedure

Through the administration of the contrast agent gadolinium (Gd) which is injected into the vein, valuable additional information can be obtained in MS diagnostics, especially when making a diagnosis. Let us first take a closer look at the procedure of an MRI examination.

During the examination, the first MRI image series are performed **without** contrast medium. Only then, if necessary, is the contrast medium administered, and further image series are subsequently added. The contrast medium containing gadolinium cannot normally pass through the blood–brain barrier due to its large molecular size and therefore cannot pass from the blood into the brain. Only in the case of an inflammation-related disturbance of the blood–brain barrier (e.g. in the context of an MS relapse) can the contrast medium overcome this barrier and enter the brain. There, it leads to increased signalling in the regions **freshly** affected by inflammation, so that these regions light up brightly in the MRI image.

> Brightly illuminated lesions in the MRI after contrast medium administration thus indicate acute inflammation in these brain regions and are an indication of a disturbance of the blood–brain barrier, because otherwise the contrast medium could not have reached the brain.

4.6.2   T1-Weighted Images: Fresh Acute MS Lesions Particularly Visible

For the assessment of the gadolinium effect, the T1-weighted MRI images are of particular importance. In the presentation of the image contrasts, we had already asked ourselves why T1 images are actually taken when no MS lesions can usually be seen at all in T1. Here comes the answer: because MS lesions are usually **not visible at all** in the T1 image or are **darker** than the

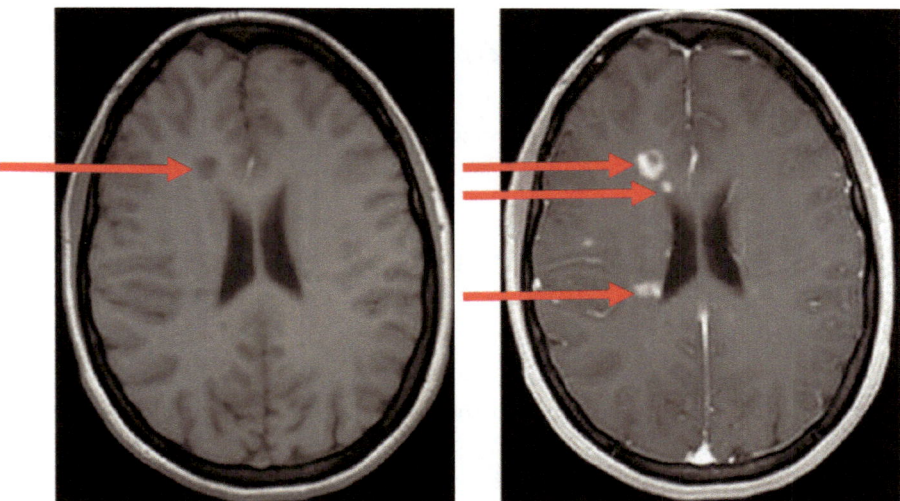

Fig. 4.16 Fresh MS lesions in T1 MRI image: left before and right after gadolinium administration

surrounding brain tissue, the fresh gadolinium-positive lesions, which are brightly illuminated by the contrast medium, stand out particularly strongly in T1 and can be very well distinguished from the dark brain tissue (Fig. 4.16).

The figure shows a T1-weighted image **before** (left) and **after** (right) the administration of gadolinium. In the left image, you can see only one lesion in the white matter, which is dark (hypointense). As already mentioned, we cannot make any statement about the number of MS lesions in T1-weighted images, because the lesions can look the same as the brain tissue (isointense) and are therefore not recognisable. The right image shows the same MRI slice, but now **after** the administration of gadolinium. The previously dark, hypointense area appears bright after the administration of contrast medium, and two further lesions are also shown, which were not visible at all without the contrast medium. These three lesions in the right MRI image, which light up brightly after the administration of contrast medium, are new, inflammatory lesions that indicate a blood–brain barrier disorder. But what does "new" actually mean?

4.6.3 Age Determination of MS Lesions Possible Thanks to Contrast Agent

The contrast behaviour of inflammatory altered regions changes over time. While at the beginning of the inflammation fresh lesions light up brightly and show a strong, ring-shaped or flat contrast medium signal, the lesions fade over time and become smaller. After 8–12 weeks, they are either no longer visible in the T1 images (isointense) or they leave a dark spot (hypointense).

> Due to this temporally changing contrast behaviour, new lesions that have developed in the last 2–3 months can be distinguished from older lesions.

4.6.4   Early Diagnosis Thanks to Contrast Agent

The chronology of the appearance of the lesions is particularly important in the diagnosis of MS, because after the appearance of the first symptoms in a suspected MS, we need evidence of the diagnostic criterion "dissemination in time" (DIT) (Sect. 2.1).

After the **first clinical episode** with evidence of several MS-suspicious lesions in the MRI, the diagnosis of MS can be made if new lesions are found in the MRI at the same time as older ones. In this case, the MRI provides evidence and ensures that the MS diagnosis can be made at an early stage, even before a possible second relapse.

> The T1-weighted MRI images without, and then in comparison with, contrast medium are therefore used to detect new lesions that have developed in the last 2–3 months. This shows the dissemination in time and allows for an early diagnosis of MS because dissemination in time is one of the important diagnostic criteria for MS (Sect. 4.8).

4.7   "Black Holes", "Footprints", Brain Atrophy: And What They Mean

We have discussed what happens to a new, inflammatory lesion over time: It heals with scarring. In the following, we will take a closer look at what healing looks like in the MRI. Here, too, we have to differentiate between the T1 and the T2 MRI images, because both show the healing process differently (Fig. 4.17).

4.7.1   The Healing Process After Acute Inflammation: Black Holes and Footprints

While in T2-weighted MRIs even old lesions remain visible as bright spots (Fig. 4.17, bottom row), they can no longer be detected at all in the T1 image (Fig. 4.17, upper line right image, marked with arrow) or they heal as a dark

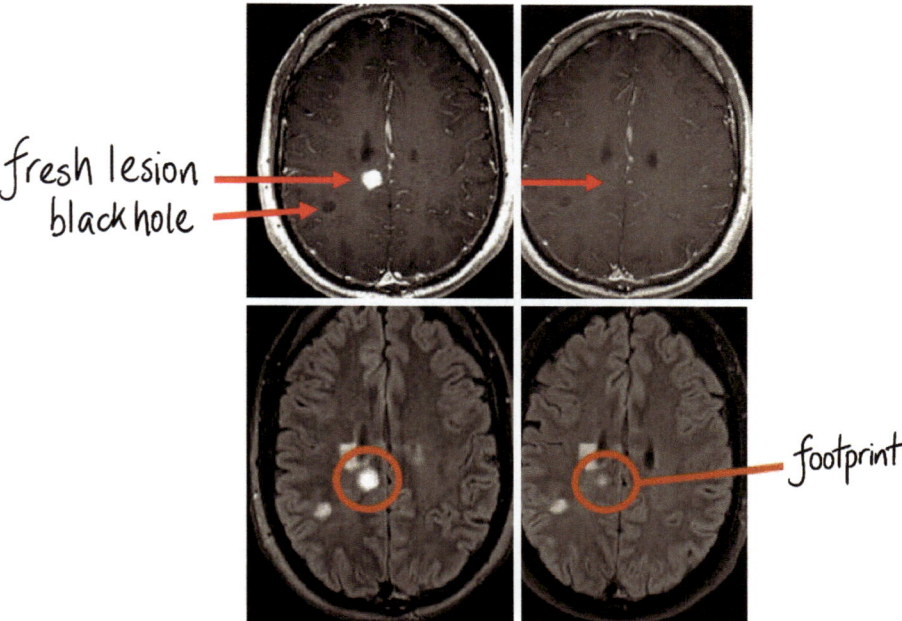

fresh lesion
black hole

footprint

Fig. 4.17 Contrast behaviour of a fresh lesion over time (after month 1 and month 3). Top row, T1 image with contrast medium: the lesion is no longer detectable after 3 months. Bottom row, T2-FLAIR image: the lesion remains visible as a footprint even after 3 months

spot. These dark spots in T1, which do not absorb any contrast medium even after gadolinium administration, are called "black holes" in technical jargon (Fig. 4.17: upper row, left image, marked with an arrow).

> A "black hole" in T1 with contrast agent therefore corresponds to a scarred residual state of a previously active lesion. A "black hole" stands for axon loss, i.e. nerve tissue destruction.

In T2-weighted MRI images, on the other hand, all lesions—regardless of age—appear as typical "white spots" (Fig. 4.17, bottom row).

> Healed, older lesions remain in the T2 images as a kind of "footprint", hence the term "footprint" [Fig. 4.17 (●: bottom row, right image, outlined)].

Increasing scarring with footprints and black holes should of course be avoided if possible. The black holes in particular represent axon loss, i.e. the loss of nerve cells. An increasing loss of nerve cells in turn leads to a reduction in brain volume, which is also called brain atrophy. We will look at how this brain atrophy appears in the MRI in the following.

4.7.2   When the Brain Changes: Brain Atrophy

There are many causes for a decrease in brain volume (brain atrophy). In MS, it is caused by increasing autoimmune inflammatory processes in the white matter and the cerebral cortex with cell death and scarring. In the MRI, brain atrophy is best seen in the axial layers (Fig. 4.18). It manifests itself in a certain flattening and "plumping" of the cerebral convolutions, as a result of which the outer furrows appear deeper and wider, which is also called "outer atrophy". With increasing loss of the axons in the white matter with degradation of the white matter, there is a widening of the cerebral ventricles, which is called "internal atrophy". In the T2-weighted MRI images, the lesion areas appear bright and in the T1-weighted they appear dark, as many converging black holes lying next to each other (Fig. 4.18, T2 on the left, T1 on the right). The therapeutic goal today is to avoid such a development.

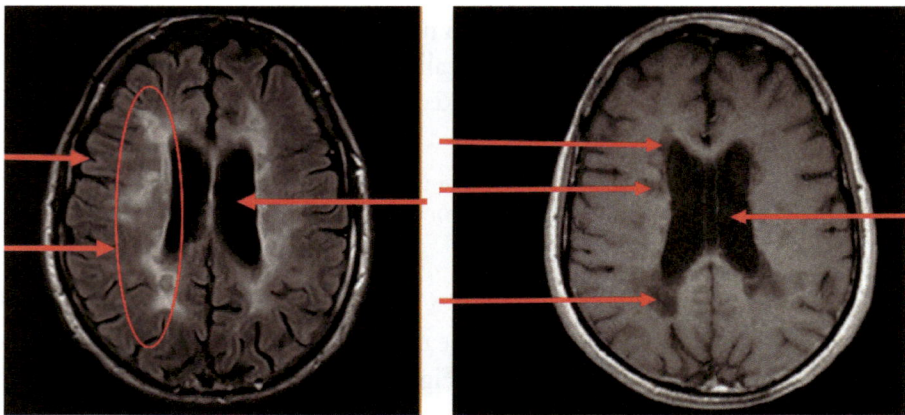

Fig. 4.18   Brain atrophy in axial section in T2-FLAIR (left) and T1 (right)

4.8   When an MRI Is Necessary: The "MRI for Diagnosis" and the "Follow-Up MRI"

As you now know, not every "white spot" in the white matter of the brain leads to a diagnosis of MS. Several factors have to be taken into account. These include the appearance of the lesions and their distribution pattern (Sect. 4.3) and the contrast behaviour of the lesions (Sect. 4.6). In order to diagnose MS, clear criteria are required, such as dissemination in space and dissemination in time (Sect. 2.1). We will look at these again in more detail from the MRI aspect in this chapter.

4.8.1   The MRI for Diagnosis

The MRI has become particularly important in the diagnosis of MS because it can provide evidence of both dissemination in space and dissemination in time in a single MRI image, which then leads to an early diagnosis of MS.

According to the diagnostic criteria for MS, the criterion of dissemination in space is fulfilled if at least two T2 lesions are found in at least two of the four typical MS locations. Typical locations are periventricular, juxtacortical, infratentorial or spinal locations (Sect. 4.3). The criterion of dissemination in time is fulfilled if new, contrast-absorbing lesions can be detected in one and the same MRI next to older, non-contrast-absorbing lesions.

If, however, no new lesions are found next to older ones in the first MRI, the dissemination in time is lacking and the diagnosis of MS cannot be made. The criterion of dissemination in time is only fulfilled if new or enlarging T2 lesions are found in a follow-up MRI.

This is illustrated once again in the following MRI image.

The first image (Fig. 4.19) shows a T2 image (left) with several typical MS lesions, thus fulfilling the criterion of dissemination in space. The lesions are oval to round; they are hyperintense in T2, i.e. bright, and are located periventricular and juxtacortical. It is not possible to distinguish between new and old lesions in these T2-weighted images alone. This is only possible by supplementing with T1-weighted images after contrast medium administration (Fig. 4.19, right). This is because the T1 image with gadolinium (right) clearly shows that **one** single lesion is bright after contrast medium administration and can therefore be considered as new. The T1 image thus makes it possible to classify the time of origin of the lesion, because this single lesion must have

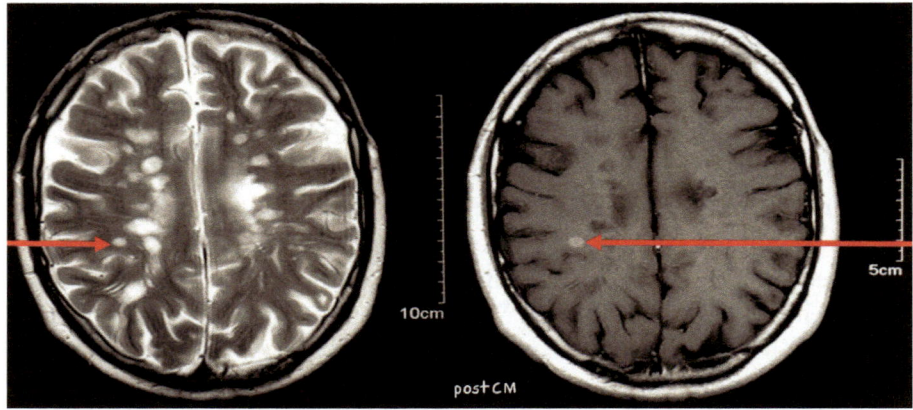

Fig. 4.19 T2 and T1 + Gd. Many lesions in T2 (left image) including one single contrast-absorbing new lesion in T1 (right image)

developed in the last 2–3 months. Therefore, in this MRI example, not only the criterion of dissemination in space but also that of dissemination in time is fulfilled and the MS diagnosis can be made according to MRI criteria.

In the second example (Fig. 4.20), you can see a follow-up MRI in T2-PD representation. The MRI on the right shows two new lesions in the white matter (marked in red) over time compared to the left. In this way, the dissemination in time can also be demonstrated by a follow-up MRI. Thus, in this MRI example, in addition to the criterion of dissemination in space, that of dissemination in time is also fulfilled and the MS diagnosis can be made.

The MRI therefore plays a very important role in the diagnosis of MS. However, an MRI is indispensable not only for making a diagnosis, but also for monitoring the course of the disease and for therapy control.

4.8.2   The MRI for Follow-Up

The MRI also plays an important role in monitoring therapy and controlling the course of the disease. Because MS can also progress without showing itself in the form of clinical relapses, we need the MRI as a progression parameter to be able to detect possible subclinical disease activity (see iceberg model from Chap. 1).

> A worsening in the control MRI under an existing therapy with new lesions is to be evaluated as progression of the disease even without the occurrence of clinical relapses!

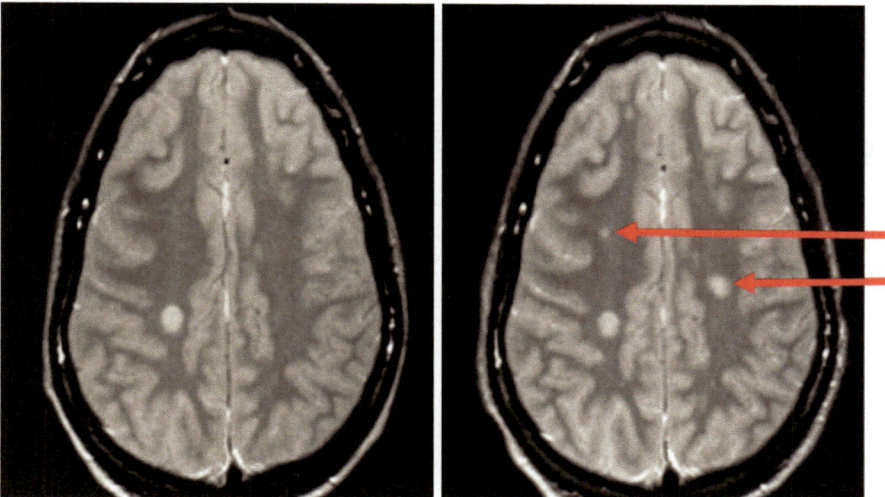

Fig. 4.20 MRI follow-up in T2-PD: one MS lesion on the left, two new lesions on the right over time

This **subclinical** worsening means that the currently existing therapy is not sufficient to suppress the inflammatory activity. In this case, a change of therapy should be considered.

The MRI as follow-up is therefore important to detect the progression of the disease at an early stage.

> Progression of MS on the MRI can be seen by new or enlarging T2 lesions or new contrast-absorbing lesions on T1-weighted MRI images.

An **MRI check** of the brain during MS therapy is nowadays usually carried out **once a year**. However, there may be individual deviations from this, depending on the type of therapy and the patient's condition. In recent years, there has been a tendency to dispense with contrast medium during the follow-up MRI. The background to this idea is that every new lesion would have absorbed contrast medium if the lesion had been captured on the MRI at the right time. The administration of contrast medium is therefore actually only necessary if explicit information is needed as to whether the lesion appeared in the last 2–3 months.

Now that we have gained a lot of knowledge about the MRI in MS, in the following chapter, we will look at typical MRIs in MS. You can apply and repeat everything you have read in the previous MRI chapters. For repetition, the sectional planes, image contrast and description of the lesions are added to each MRI image.

4.9 Typical MRI Images in MS

Now that the technical basics have been discussed in detail, we can look at a selection of MRI images typical of MS. In each case, the sectional plane, image contrast and, if applicable, contrast agent behaviour are indicated for all images and the important changes are marked with a red arrow. Here we go.

4.9.1 Corpus Callosum Lesions

See Figs. 4.21 and 4.22.

4.9.2 Brainstem Lesions

See Fig. 4.23.

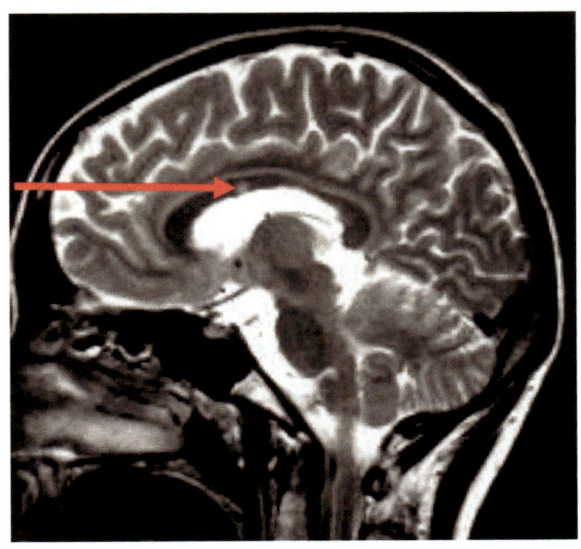

Fig. 4.21 Sagittal section, image contrast: T2 (CSF light; lesion light), typical hyperintense MS lesion in corpus callosum

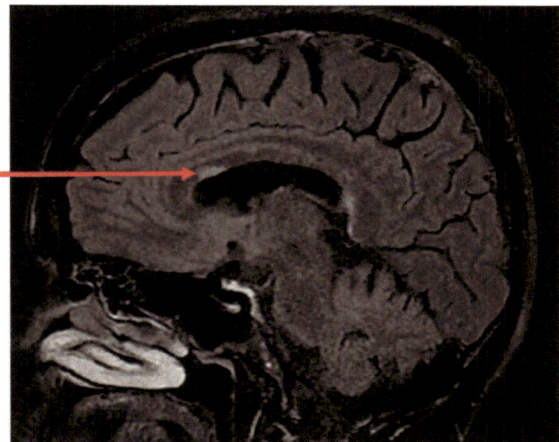

Fig. 4.22 Sagittal section. Image contrast: T2-FLAIR (CSF dark; lesion light), typical hyperintense MS lesion in corpus callosum

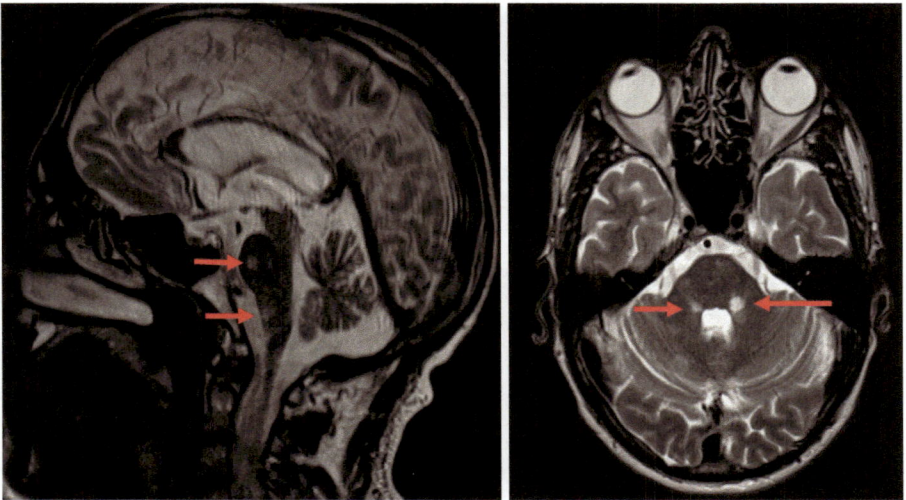

Fig. 4.23 Sagittal section (left), axial (right), image contrast: T2 (CSF light, lesions light), multiple brainstem lesions

4.9.3   Cock's Comb-Like White Matter Lesions, Also Called "Dawson Fingers"

Dawson fingers are oval lesions in the white matter aligned with the ventricle, which look like a "cock's comb" in the sagittal image. This structure is due to the fact that the inflammatory lesions of MS are aligned with the veins leading to the ventricles. In the axial layers, these lesions also look oval and are oriented towards the ventricle (Fig. 4.24).

4.9.4   Black Holes

Black holes (Fig. 4.25) are scars. Lesions that appear as black holes in T1 after administration of contrast medium, i.e. that do **not** absorb contrast medium, are referred to as "black holes". A black hole is an expression of axonal damage with nerve tissue destruction.

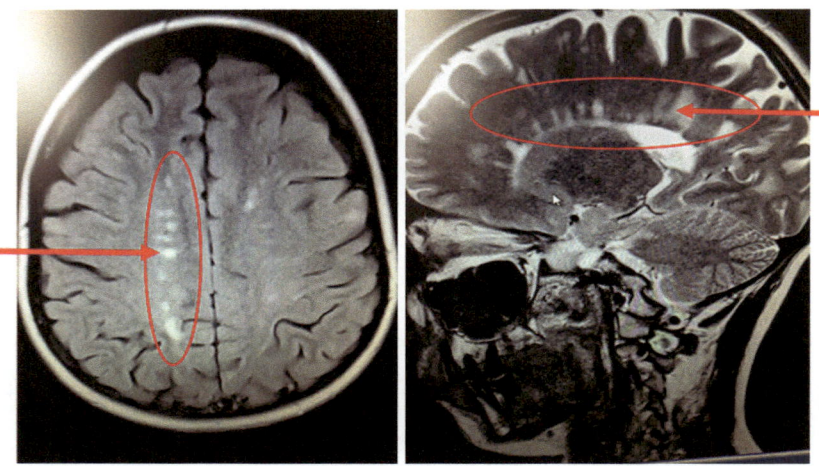

Fig. 4.24 Axial (left) and sagittal (right) sectioning, image contrast: T2-FLAIR (left) and T2 (right), typical "cock's comb-like MS lesions" or also called Dawson fingers

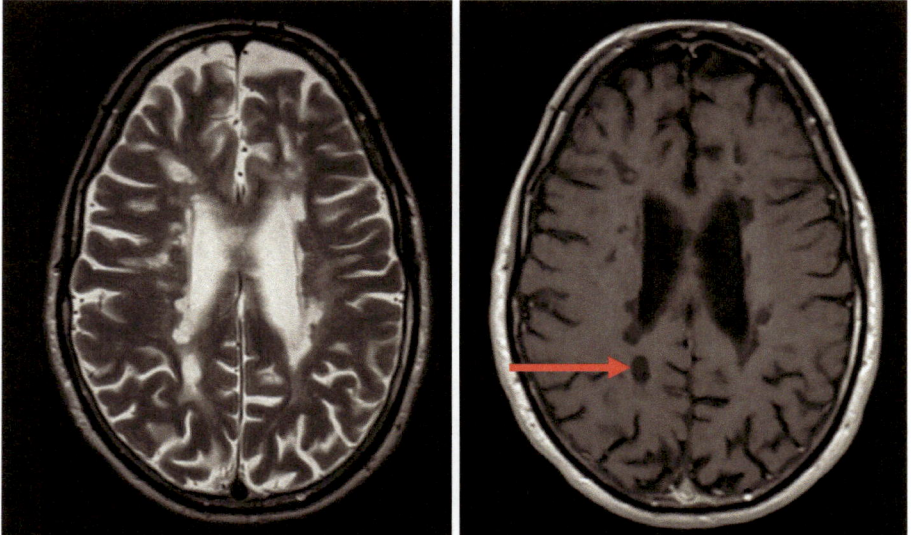

Fig. 4.25 Axial sectioning, image contrast: T2 (left), T1 + contrast medium (right), right arrow marks a black hole in the white matter

4.9.5 New Contrast-Absorbing Lesions (Fig. 4.26)

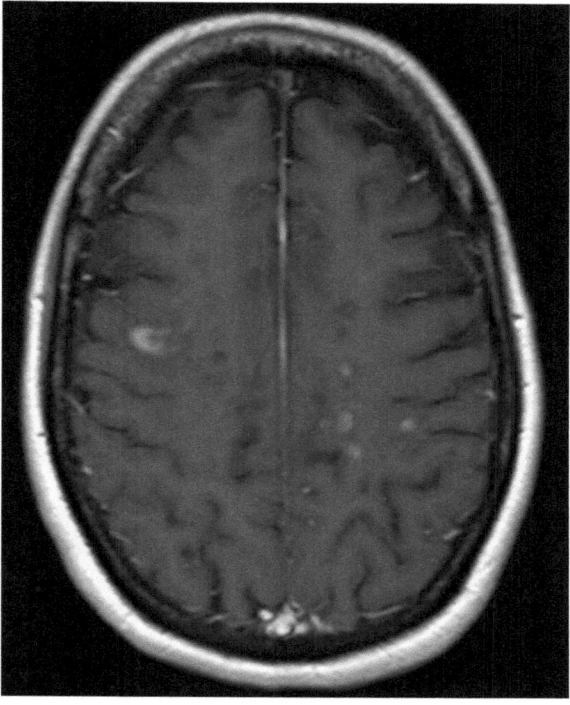

Fig. 4.26 Axial sectioning, image contrast: T1 + contrast medium, several new lesions in the white matter of different sizes, spot-shaped and also half-ring-shaped, absorbing contrast medium

4.9.6   Lesion in the Cervical Spinal Cord (Fig. 4.27)

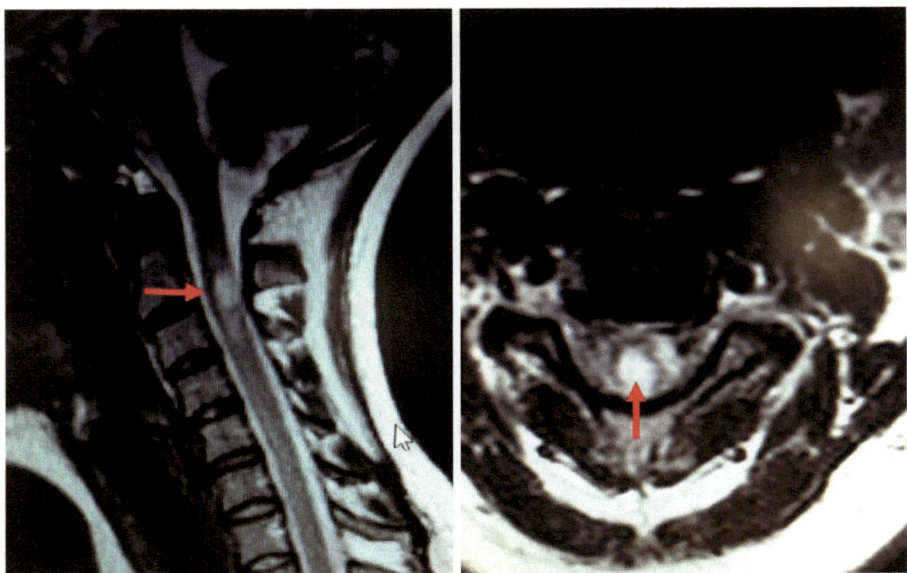

Fig. 4.27 Sagittal section (left), axial section (right), image contrast: T2 (CSF light, lesion light), large hyperintense lesion in the cervical spinal cord, occupying almost the entire spinal cord cross section

4.9.7   Brain Atrophy (Fig. 4.28)

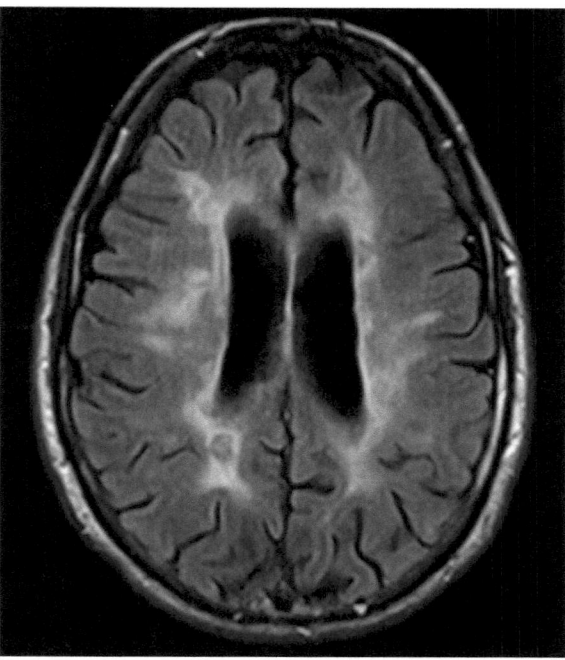

Fig. 4.28   Axial section, image contrast: T2-FLAIR (CSF dark, lesions light), large defects periventricular in the brain, and dilated ventricular system ("internal and external brain atrophy")

4.9.8   The MRI Report: *Not* a Closed Book!

Now you have got to know a wide range of MS-typical changes in the MRI and if you re-read the report again, you will be surprised how much you now understand! The MRI findings are **no** longer a closed book!

Magnetic resonance imaging of the skull with and without contrast medium from (date).

"*For comparison, an external preliminary examination dated (date) is available. Evidence of numerous patchy, partly converging signal elevations, **cockscomb like** at **corpus callosum level**, in the **periventricular white matter** and **juxta-cortically** in the **T2 and T2-FLAIR sequence.** Suspicion of a small lesion on the right **cerebellar** side. The lesions are defined as **hypointense** lesions in the **native T1 sequence.** No evidence of **pathological contrast enhancement**. Somewhat accentuated inner and outer CSF spaces. As far as can be compared with the previous images, no significant change in findings compared to the previous findings*".

Now that we have dealt with the MRI in great detail, all that is missing to perfect your diagnostic knowledge is the cerebrospinal fluid examination. And this is what we will cover in the next chapter.

5

The Most Important Things About the Cerebrospinal Fluid

5.1 Basics of the Cerebrospinal Fluid

The extraction of the cerebrospinal fluid is called lumbar puncture (LP). But what is cerebrospinal fluid and why is it so important to examine the cerebrospinal fluid in suspected MS? In order for you to better understand the findings of the cerebrospinal fluid examination in the discharge letter, we will have a closer look at "the most important things about the cerebrospinal fluid" in this chapter. This way you can see which parameters can be examined and what conclusions can be drawn from them.

5.1.1 Cerebrospinal Fluid: What It Is and Where It Comes From

The cerebrospinal fluid is the fluid that surrounds the brain and spinal cord and hydraulically protects them against shocks. Important information about the central nervous system (CNS) can be obtained from the examination of the cerebrospinal fluid (CSF).

The human body contains about 4000–6000 mL of blood, but only 120–200 mL of cerebrospinal fluid. Unlike blood, cerebrospinal fluid is a clear, colourless liquid that contains much less protein and cells than blood. The cerebrospinal fluid is formed in special cells in the so-called choroid plexus in the ventricles (brain chambers) of the brain. About 500 mL is produced per day, and the same amount is reabsorbed into the bloodstream.

5.1.2   Blood and Cerebrospinal Fluid: Two Separate Areas

The cerebrospinal fluid passes through the blood–brain barrier (BBB, Fig. 5.1) from the bloodstream. This barrier is formed by blood capillary cells, known as endothelial cells.

> The blood–brain barrier consists of a single-row cell layer, the endothelium, which lies on the inside of the brain vessels and is only permeable to very specific substances.

This blood–brain barrier (BBB) prevents the exchange between blood and CSF so they cannot mix, so the composition of the two fluids is **not** identical.

> Because the composition of blood and CSF is not identical due to the separation of the two areas by the blood–brain barrier (BBB), a blood examination cannot replace the CSF examination, but must complement it!

Similar to a sieve, the permeability of the blood–brain barrier is primarily determined by the size of the molecule. Only dissolved substances or very small molecules can normally pass through the barrier. In the case of inflammatory CNS diseases, the permeability of the blood–brain barrier changes, so

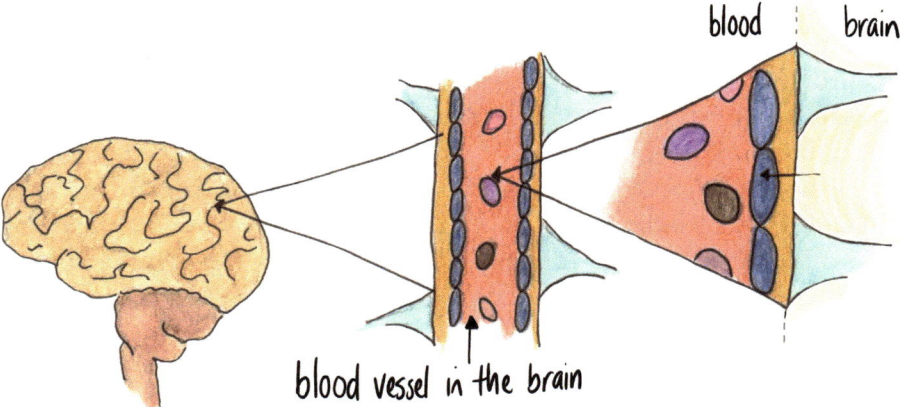

Fig. 5.1   The blood–brain barrier

that larger particles, such as larger cells or, for example, the contrast medium in MRI examinations, can pass through the barrier and enter the brain.

To reduce any fears and uncertainty before the lumbar puncture (LP), I would like to briefly describe how the lumbar puncture is performed in the next chapter.

5.2   How a Lumbar Puncture Works

The decision as to whether a lumbar puncture (LP) should be performed under outpatient or inpatient conditions must be made on an individual basis. Much more decisive is the rapid and professional forwarding of the freshly obtained cerebrospinal fluid and the prompt processing of the CSF in the laboratory. The transport must not be delayed because otherwise there is a risk of cell dissolution, which can lead to misjudgements. It is also important that CSF and blood are always taken at the same time, as the comparison of the two is crucial for the interpretation of the findings.

5.2.1   Practical Procedure

The lumbar puncture can be done lying down or sitting up. The puncture site is in the lower back between the third and fourth or also fourth and fifth lumbar vertebrae. The puncture through the skin is similar to a blood sample. The skin is carefully cleaned locally with a disinfectant spray beforehand. A very fine, thin needle is used to quickly reach the spinal canal and the cerebrospinal fluid space. Approximately 10–15 mL of the CSF (normally as transparent as water) is taken for examination purposes.

The exact evaluation of the cerebrospinal fluid is described in the next chapter. It is important to mention that the widespread term "spinal cord puncture" is factually incorrect because, as you have already read (Sect. 1.3), the spinal cord ends at the level of the first lumbar vertebra. At the puncture height L3/4 or 4/5, there is therefore no spinal cord left and it cannot be injured.

5.2.2   After That …

In order to avoid so-called post-puncture headaches, i.e. headaches that can occur in up to 5% of people after a CSF puncture, it is important to follow a few rules after the puncture. If you think of a blood sample, you probably remember that you have to press on the puncture site with a swab a little longer afterwards to prevent the blood from running further. In the case of a lumbar puncture, this "squeezing" is done a little differently: you should **lie on your stomach for half an hour to an hour** *after* the puncture to prevent the blood from dripping, because then the puncture canal closes more quickly. But it also makes sense to lie down as much as possible for the rest of the day.

5.3   What the Lumbar Puncture Tells Us: The Evaluation

In this chapter, we will see what is examined in the cerebrospinal fluid, what information we can get from the result of the lumbar puncture and what the "typical" MS changes in the cerebrospinal fluid look like. You will find these findings in the discharge letter.

Lumbar puncture is mainly used to detect inflammatory processes in the CNS, and it gives indications of functional disorders of the blood–brain barrier. It plays a major role in differentiating MS from other diseases, especially those that can produce the same symptoms or similar MRI changes. Here, for example, the tick-borne Lyme disease should be mentioned, which in rare cases can also affect the CNS as so-called neuroborreliosis. However, vascular or rheumatic diseases can also affect the CNS and must be differentiated from MS.

5.3.1   The CSF Examination: Cell Count, Total Protein, Sugar and Lactate

The examination of the CSF begins with the so-called "cytology". Here, the number of cells per µL in the CSF is examined; however, not only the pure number of cells is important, but also the type of cells in the CSF is of interest. In this way, a distinction can be made as to whether lymphocytes are mainly detectable—as is typical for MS—or whether other cells such as granulocytes are predominant (Chap. 3), which is typical in bacterial CNS infections.

In addition to the cell count, the total protein as well as the sugar and lactate content in the cerebrospinal fluid are always measured during the CSF examination. These four parameters alone can often distinguish infectious diseases caused by bacteria or viruses from autoimmune diseases such as MS.

In addition to these described parameters, you can also read terms such as "albumin quotient", "intrathecal immunoglobulin synthesis" and "oligoclonal

> While a significant increase in cell count, protein and lactate with a drop in glucose (i.e. sugar) in the CSF is typical for infectious diseases, these values are often inconspicuous in MS.

bands" in the CSF findings. As we will see in a moment, these three values provide information about the blood–brain barrier function and about a possible autoimmune process in the central nervous system itself.

5.3.2 Blood–Brain Barrier Function: Albumin Shows What Is Going On

How can you tell that the BBB is dense? To understand this, we first need to familiarise ourselves with albumin. Albumin is a **large** protein and serves as evidence of a functioning blood–brain barrier. Why? Albumin is only produced outside the brain, namely in the liver, and because of its size, it cannot pass through the blood–brain barrier! Because, as we have heard, the permeability of the blood–brain barrier is determined by the size of the molecule. Albumin, as a large protein, **cannot** pass the barrier under normal conditions. It therefore only occurs in the blood and not in the cerebrospinal fluid.

> Albumin detectable in the CSF can therefore only come from the blood and thus speaks for a "leaky barrier".

5.3.3 The Albumin Quotient

The determination of albumin in CSF and blood and the relationship to each other is expressed by the so-called albumin quotient (QAlb) (calculated according to QAlb = albumin concentration in CSF/albumin concentration in serum).

> A high albumin quotient therefore indicates the detection of albumin in the CNS and thus an increased permeability of the blood–brain barrier. The albumin quotient QAlb is thus the decisive value for the functional assessment of the blood–brain barrier.

5.3.4   Antibodies Made in the CNS Itself: The IgG Quotient

In addition to albumin, other proteins in the CSF and serum are examined and compared to each other, e.g. the immunoglobulins IgG, IgA and IgM. These immunoglobulins of different sizes are antibodies formed by plasma cells, which you already know about from Chap. 3, "A Trip into Our Immune System".

> The concentration of the various immunoglobulins in the CSF depends on their size, their concentration in the blood and, of course, also the blood–brain barrier function.

Just as with albumin, a quotient can be formed in the same way for the individual immunoglobulins; this describes the immunoglobulin ratio of CSF to blood. Since the immunoglobulins G (IgG) are particularly important for MS diagnostics, we will limit ourselves to these in the following and look at the IgG and the IgG quotient (QIgG) (calculated according to QIgG = IgG concentration in the CSF/IgG concentration in the serum). If the IgG quotient is elevated, we must assume that either the IgGs detected in the CSF originate from the blood and have been able to cross the barrier in greater numbers or they have been produced in the central nervous system itself, which is then called "intrathecal IgG production".

> Intrathecal IgG production, i.e. IgG made in the CNS itself, is typical for MS.

5.3.5   The Reiber Diagram

For the analysis of these immunoglobulins in the cerebrospinal fluid, the German biochemist Professor Reiber developed a quotient diagram with a graphic representation of the quotients to make the whole thing clearer. This diagram is accordingly called the Reiber diagram. By plotting the albumin quotient against the immunoglobulin quotients, typical constellations of findings can be easily read at a glance, as you will see later. Here, too, we will limit ourselves in the following to the diagram for IgG, since IgA and IgM play a minor role in the MS diagnostics.

Since these diagrams are sometimes also found in the discharge report, we want to look at practical examples of how they are read and interpreted.

Fig. 5.2 The Reiber diagram, CSF/serum quotient diagram for IgG. (Graphical representation of the quotients of Reiber and Felgenhauer)

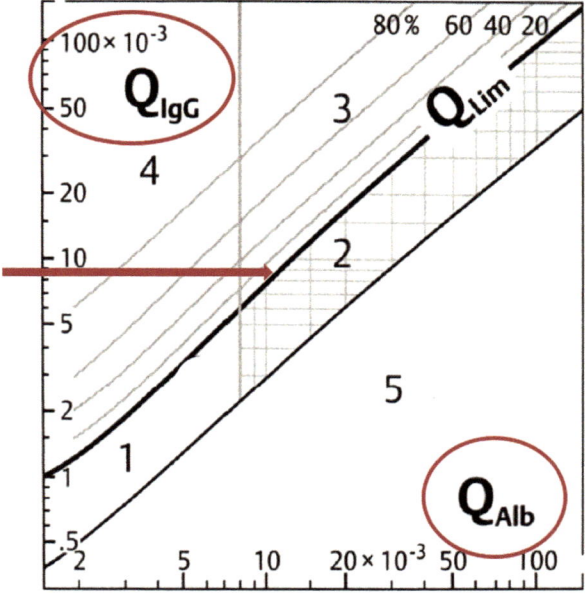

In the Reiber diagram for IgG, the albumin quotient (QAlb) and the IgG quotient (QIgG) are related to each other. From their ratio, it can be read graphically whether it is a blood–brain barrier disorder or an intrathecal IgG production or both.

In the Reiber diagram, you will find the albumin quotient (QAlb) plotted on the horizontal axis (*x*-axis) and the IgG quotient (QIgG) plotted on the vertical axis (*y*-axis) of the diagram (Fig. 5.2, marked in red).

5.3.6 Deviations Upwards on the Vertical: Too Much IgG in the CSF

A thick line rising from the lower left to the upper right is conspicuous (Fig. 5.2, marked with a red arrow). This bold line (Q Lim) represents the upper limit of the normal range of the albumin/IgG ratio.

Values below the borderline indicate normal findings. Values above the line, on the other hand, indicate too much IgG in the CSF, and thus, IgG was produced in the CNS itself (intrathecal IgG), which would be an expression of an autoimmune process in the CNS.

This so-called intrathecal IgG production is typical for MS. In the diagram, you can see four more thin dashed lines above the bold line. They allow you to estimate the extent of intrathecal IgG production in % (i.e. 20%, 40%, 60% or 80% above the upper limit of the normal range).

5.3.7 Deviations to the Right on the Horizontal Axis: Too Much Albumin in the CSF

Now we look at the horizontal axis with the albumin quotient (QAlb) (Fig. 5.3). It gives us information about the amount of albumin in the CSF and thus about the blood–brain barrier function. Since the albumin quotient is age-dependent, the age-adjusted quotient is first entered as a vertical line in the diagram (Fig. 5.3: "20/40/60 years", marked by red line at 60 years).

All values to **the left of** the vertical, age-adapted line indicate normal findings and correspond to a functioning, "tight" blood–brain barrier. All readings to the right of this line indicate too high albumin levels in the CSF and thus a blood–brain barrier disorder—the further to the right, the more pronounced the barrier disorder.

Fig. 5.3 The Reiber diagram: assessing blood–brain barrier function

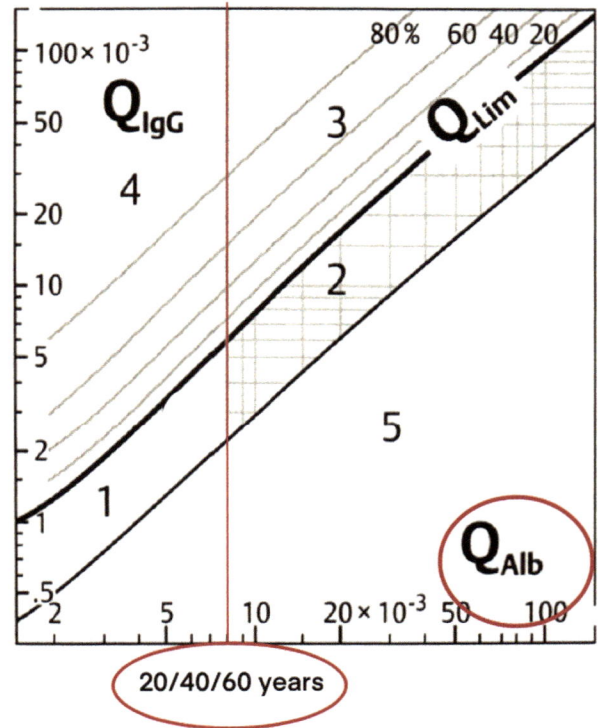

5.3.8   And Now a Few Examples: The Normal Finding

Now that you have learned about the structure and interpretation of the Reiber diagram, let us look at three different cases: a normal finding and two possible MS constellations. Let us start with the Reiber diagram of a normal finding (Fig. 5.4).

The red measurement point lies to **the left of the** vertical line of the age-dependent albumin quotient and thus indicates an intact blood–brain barrier function. The measured value is also **below the** bold line marking the upper normal range of the albumin/IgG quotient. This means that there is **no** indication of intrathecal immunoglobulin G production. This is what a normal result looks like in the Reiber diagram.

5.3.9   MS-Typical Findings: Intrathecal IgG Production

In the following second example, things look different (Fig. 5.5): The measured value entered in red is again to **the left of** the reference value for the age-dependent albumin quotient and thus, as in the previous example,

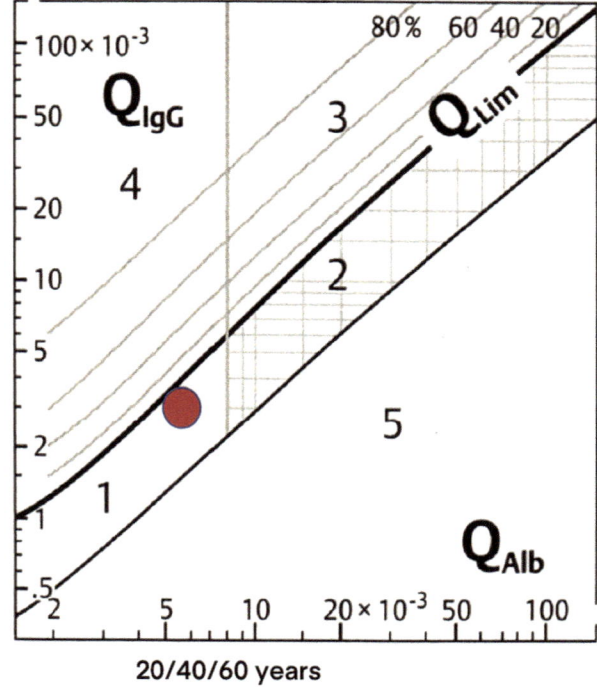

Fig. 5.4 Reiber diagram: normal findings

Fig. 5.5 Reiber diagram:
intrathecal IgG
production

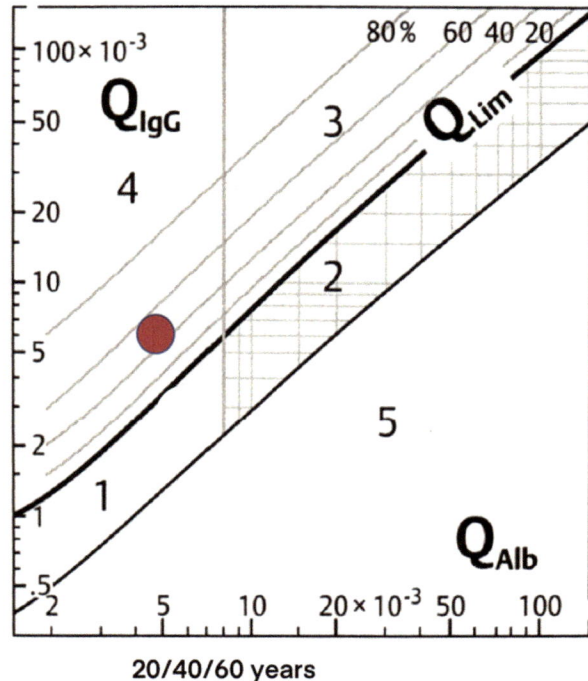

20/40/60 years

indicates an intact blood–brain barrier function. However, the value entered in red is now **above the** bold line. The finding thus indicates increased IgG in the CSF in relation to the blood and thus indicates that the IgG must have originated in the central nervous system itself, i.e. independently of the blood. This finding corresponds to a typical MS finding with the so-called intrathecal IgG production.

5.3.10 Another MS-Typical Constellation

The following example also shows a constellation that is possible with the MS (Fig. 5.6). The value entered in red is again **above the** line printed in bold and thus indicates intrathecal IgG production. However, the measured value entered in red now also lies to **the right of** the reference value for the age-dependent albumin quotient in the range indicating a blood–brain barrier disorder. This finding is also a typical MS finding that, in addition to intrathecal IgG production, also indicates a disturbed blood–brain barrier function.

Now that you have become familiar with terms such as "albumin quotient" and "intrathecal immunoglobulin synthesis", there is only one last, but very

Fig. 5.6 Reiber diagram: intrathecal IgG production and blood–brain barrier dysfunction

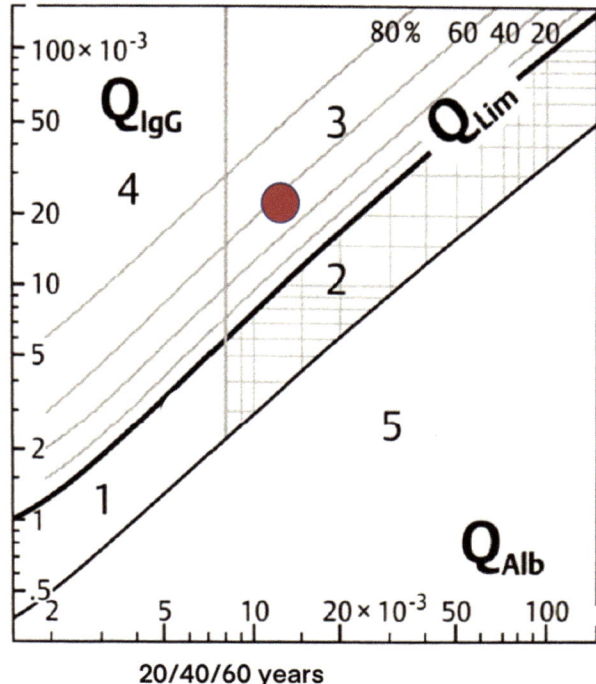

20/40/60 years

important value missing in the CSF diagnosis of MS: the so-called "oligoclonal bands", also abbreviated OCB.

5.3.11   Isoelectric Focusing and Oligoclonal Bands (OCBs)

The detection of intrathecal IgG production in MS is also possible by another method that is even more sensitive than quotient formation. This method is called isoelectric focusing. Here, serum (serum is the liquid part of the blood that is obtained as supernatant when blood is centrifuged) and CSF are applied separately on a kind of blotting paper (Fig. 5.7). An electrical voltage is then applied to the paper, and the negatively charged protein molecules migrate in the voltage field to different extents towards the positive pole of the blotting paper. The protein molecules, which included the various immunoglobulins, are separated in this way and are detectable as different "bands" on the paper. These bands are called oligoclonal bands (OCBs).

If isoelectric focusing shows bands that only occur in the CSF, but not in the serum (blood), this is an indication of IgG produced in the CNS itself (intrathecal IgG production) and thus evidence of an autoimmune process in the CNS (Fig. 5.7).

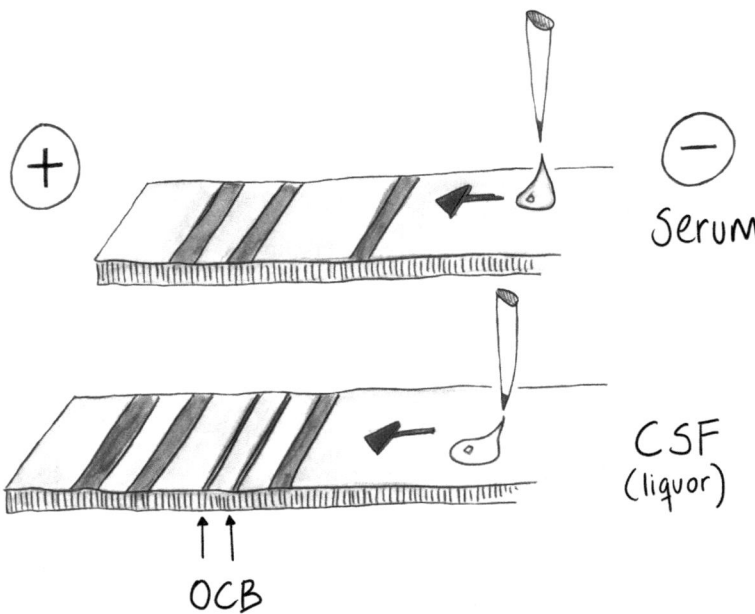

Fig. 5.7 Isoelectric focusing and oligoclonal bands

It is therefore always necessary to compare serum (blood) and CSF in order to obtain a statement. Although one speaks of "positive OCB", one should correctly say: "the OCBs for IgG are positive in the CSF and negative in the serum". This finding is typical for MS.

However, the OCBs are not specific for a disease pattern and not for MS either, because they can also be positive in other inflammatory diseases of the CNS. They only show that an inflammatory process in the central nervous system takes place independently of the blood. However, the OCBs are more sensitive than the quotient diagram for the detection of intrathecal IgG production.

Although the OCBs are detectable in the CSF in 88–98% of MS cases, they can still be negative, especially at the beginning of the MS disease. However, the probability of their detection increases with the amount of inflammatory lesions present in the CNS and the length of the course of the disease.

In this detailed chapter on cerebrospinal fluid, you have now learned a lot about CSF examination, blood–brain barrier analysis, detection of intrathecal immunoglobulin synthesis using the Reiber diagram and isoelectric focusing. With this information, you can now review and better assess findings.

Now that we have dealt in detail with the MS disease, the diagnosis, the autoimmune process and the necessary examinations—especially the MRI and the lumbar puncture—in Part I of the book, the following Part II of the book focuses on MS therapy.

Part II

MS: Understanding the Therapy

6

How MS Is Treated

When we talk about MS therapy, we basically have to distinguish between two therapies:

1. First, there is the **relapse therapy** of MS. This is the acute treatment given during the MS relapse when new symptoms have developed.
2. Furthermore, there is the so-called **immunomodulatory, disease-modifying therapy**. This is the therapy that positively influences the chronic course of the disease and is intended to prevent new symptoms or increasing disability later in the course of the disease.

While the relapse therapy of MS is quickly described, there are now many different options for the disease-modifying therapy. We will take a closer look at both the acute therapy and the disease-modifying therapy in the following chapters.

Let us first start with the therapy of the acute MS relapse, which is usually carried out with cortisone.

© The Author(s), under exclusive license to Springer-Verlag GmbH, DE, part of Springer Nature 2023
A. Friedrich, *The Multiple Sclerosis Companion*,
https://doi.org/10.1007/978-3-662-67540-3_6

7

What To Do in an Acute MS Attack

If a new relapse is on the horizon, i.e. new complaints appear, there is a clear recommendation, which is this:

In the case of an acute attack, see a neurologist as soon as possible!

If new symptoms appear that last longer than 24 h, it is probably an acute attack and should be treated as soon as possible. An MS relapse is treated with cortisone.

7.1 Cortisone Pulse Therapy: How Is It Done?

As a rule, the neurologist will give 1000 mg of cortisone as an infusion over 3–5 days. The total dose of this so-called cortisone pulse therapy depends on the severity of the symptoms and the tendency to regress under treatment. The cortisone pulse therapy is usually carried out in specialised MS practices on an outpatient basis. Cortisone usually leads to a rapid regression of the acute symptoms. Why? Cortisone has a strong anti-inflammatory effect because it prevents the T cells from releasing inflammatory messenger substances. In addition, cortisone seals the blood–brain barrier and interrupts the inflammatory process, because the immune cells can then no longer cross over from the blood into the CNS (Chap. 3).

© The Author(s), under exclusive license to Springer-Verlag GmbH, DE, part of Springer Nature 2023
A. Friedrich, *The Multiple Sclerosis Companion*,
https://doi.org/10.1007/978-3-662-67540-3_7

However, if the symptoms do not improve sufficiently, either a second, higher dose cortisone shot can follow or a so-called plasma exchange treatment can be carried out. Both therapy options are usually carried out as "escalation therapy of the acute relapse" under inpatient conditions, i.e. in hospital.

7.2   Plasma Exchange Treatment: Plasmapheresis and Immunoadsorption

Plasma exchange treatments, such as plasmapheresis and immunoadsorption, are necessary for severely debilitating relapses that do not respond to high-dose cortisone pulse therapy. If indicated, these treatments should be started as early as possible, but no later than 6 weeks after the start of symptoms. Both forms of therapy are reserved for specialised centres and are carried out under inpatient conditions.

In plasma exchange treatment, proteins are removed from the organism via an access into the vein. As you have already read, proteins play an important role in the autoimmune process of MS (see Part I). In plasmapheresis, the proteins are removed rather unspecifically. In contrast, immunoadsorption specifically filters the immunoglobulins, i.e. the antibodies from the blood. Plasma exchange treatments are very promising. If they are carried out early after the onset of symptoms, in up to 70% of cases, the relapse symptoms are largely or even completely reversed, so that this is an invasive (i.e. more intrusive) but very effective form of therapy.

Although cortisone pulse therapy and plasma exchange treatments usually lead to a rapid regression of the acute symptoms, there is no evidence of an effect on the relapse rate or the long-term course. For this reason, acute relapse therapy is not sufficient to suppress the disease activity of the autoimmune disease in the long-term course. This requires the so-called immunomodulatory, disease-modifying MS therapy, which we will cover in the next chapter.

8

I'm Fine: Why Therapy?

Let us be honest, how many of you affected have not asked yourselves this question? The thought process is understandable. But from the understanding of the chronic autoimmune process of MS (Chap. 3, A Trip into Our Immune System), the generally applicable therapy recommendation today is to treat every newly diagnosed MS patient as early as possible and thus ideally immediately after diagnosis. The idea is to intervene **as early as** possible. The idea is to intervene in the chronic disease process as early as possible in order to avoid the threat of disability in the future.

> So, we treat as early as possible, precisely because it is *still* going well and so that it stays that way if possible!

In the initial stage of the disease, inflammation predominates with the attack of T and B lymphocytes, plasma cells and antibodies, followed by demyelination of the nerve fibres and subsequent scarring (Chap. 3).

This process is clinically manifested by relapses, in which the symptoms often completely disappear in the beginning. This phase is called RRMS or "relapsing-remitting MS". Later on, the clinical course often changes. There may be relapses whose symptoms do **not** always completely resolve and increasing residual symptoms with disability remain. This is the transition to the chronic form of the disease, in which there are often no more clearly definable relapses, but where the symptoms increase gradually. A slowly increasing disability develops. This form is called SPMS or "secondary

© The Author(s), under exclusive license to Springer-Verlag GmbH, DE, part of Springer Nature 2023
A. Friedrich, *The Multiple Sclerosis Companion*,
https://doi.org/10.1007/978-3-662-67540-3_8

progressive MS". The slowly developing, rather insidious disability is accompanied by an increasing destruction of nerve tissue with tissue loss and brain volume reduction. And it is precisely this development that is to be prevented with the early, long-term therapy of MS!

The realisation that the initial phase of MS is characterised by acute inflammation, but the further course of MS by degeneration, i.e. degradation with increasing loss of nerve cells and scarring, is important for therapeutic understanding. Because while the first phase can be efficiently influenced by anti-inflammatory drugs, this is hardly possible in the second progressive stage. In this phase, instead of anti-inflammatory approaches, neuroreparative therapy approaches would be more necessary, i.e. therapies that could repair damaged nerve tissue. Unfortunately, such therapies do not yet exist.

> And it is precisely because we currently have no drugs to repair nerve cells that it is so important to intervene early in the disease process to preserve, if possible, what has not yet been attacked.

Statements such as "I'm fine, why therapy?" or "And if I'm not feeling well, I'll definitely come back right away!" are perhaps understandable from the patient's point of view. But, from the understanding of the chronic disease process, it becomes clear that early therapy makes sense, precisely because things are still going well!

> Early therapy exactly then when things are still going well and because things are still going well!

This information is very important. Only those who understand why early therapy makes sense can commit to the early therapy. Those who think that it makes no sense to treat complaints that are not even there are more likely to discontinue therapy.

In the following chapters, we will take a closer look at the therapeutic options. First, you will get an overview of the development of the MS therapy landscape over the last 20–25 years and learn about the different therapy concepts and how they have changed over time. You will see what criteria are used today to select an individual MS therapy and what additional considerations are taken into account. This is followed by an overview of the disease-modifying drugs currently approved for MS, also called "DMD", an abbreviation for "disease-modifying drug". What is the therapy goal and how can I tell if my therapy is working? We will deal with this in the therapy chapter, "The Therapy Goal Has a Name: NEDA".

9

MS Therapy Yesterday and Today

In this chapter, you will be guided through the jungle of immunomodulatory therapies and we start with the development of MS therapy in the 1990s. After all, modern MS therapy is not that old. Prior to that, multiple sclerosis therapy consisted mainly of trying to alleviate symptoms. Later, the aim was to **influence** the progression of the disease. Today, the therapeutic goal is to **stop** the progression of the disease. Although it is not yet possible to repair destroyed nerve tissue, it is of course the wishful thinking of the future of therapy.

9.1 Development of the MS Therapy Landscape

When I started out as a neurologist in 1998, MS therapy was still very straightforward. It mainly consisted of the medicinal treatment of symptoms such as increased muscle tension (spasticity), pain or bladder dysfunction and was characterised by physiotherapeutic, occupational therapy and speech therapy measures. Of course, these accompanying therapies and measures are still very important today, but they are rather supportive and do not influence the future course of the disease.

© The Author(s), under exclusive license to Springer-Verlag GmbH, DE, part of Springer Nature 2023
A. Friedrich, *The Multiple Sclerosis Companion*,
https://doi.org/10.1007/978-3-662-67540-3_9

9.2   Interferons and Glatiramer Acetate

In the early 1990s, the first drugs intervening with the immune process were approved, first the **interferon** beta-1b (Betaferon/Betaseron), shortly followed by the interferon beta-1a (Avonex and Rebif). There were no MS drugs before which modulated the misprogrammed immune system. In this respect, the development of interferons for MS therapy was a major milestone. As is often the case with novel therapies, it took a few years before interferons were really widely used for MS therapy. Even today, interferons are firmly established in MS treatment and are considered a very safe and effective group of substances.

In 2001, the therapeutic spectrum was expanded by another substance when **glatiramer acetate** (Copaxone) was approved, which—like all interferon preparations—also has to be injected. This provided a second therapeutic option in 2001, so that a change of therapy to another substance group was possible in case of side effects or therapy failure. Glatiramer acetate also has a wide range of applications today and, like the interferons, is considered a very effective and safe substance.

9.3   Natalizumab and Fingolimod for Escalation

In 2006, **natalizumab** (Tysabri), the first antibody therapy in MS treatment, was approved. As a highly effective drug, it is successfully used today in cases of therapy failure and in aggressive MS. Tysabri is administered as an infusion therapy every 4 weeks and has a firm place in the therapy of (highly) active MS.

Five years later, the first "MS tablet", **fingolimod** (Gilenya), was added in 2011. Fingolimod, like natalizumab, is successfully used in (highly) active MS or when a previous therapy has failed.

9.4   Alternative in Tablet Form: Teriflunomide and Dimethyl Fumarate

Since 2013, more and more new drugs have been added. With **teriflunomide** as Aubagio at the end of 2013 and **dimethyl fumarate** as Tecfidera at the beginning of 2014, two oral drugs were approved for the basic therapy of MS. This was once again a revolution in MS treatment, because for many patients for whom previously only "injection therapies" (so-called injectables) were available, there was for the first time, an alternative in tablet form in the area of basic therapy.

9.5 Long-Acting Interferon: PEG Interferon

Furthermore, the therapeutic spectrum of interferons was expanded in 2014 by the PEG interferon beta-1a as Plegridy, which has to be injected much less frequently than the previously approved interferons. Due to its large molecule size, the PEG interferon is injected subcutaneously only every 14 days instead of once or several times a week (as is usually the case with interferon therapies).

9.6 Antibody Therapies: Alemtuzumab and Ocrelizumab

Increasing knowledge about the immune system has led to more antibody therapies being used in MS treatment. These include **alemtuzumab** (Lemtrada) since 2013 and **ocrelizumab** (Ocrevus) since 2018, both approved for (highly) active MS therapy. Both are administered as infusion therapy, alemtuzumab once a year for a total of 2 years and ocrelizumab continuously every 6 months.

9.7 Cladribine: Oral Pulse Therapy

With a completely different therapeutic approach, **cladribine** (Mavenclad) was approved in 2017 for (highly) active MS, a tablet that needs to be taken as a "short-term oral treatment" only on a few days within a treatment period of 2 years.

And there are now even more therapy options since 2020 when this book was first published in German.

9.8 Siponimod Approved for SPMS

Siponimod (Mayzent) has similarities to fingolimod. But unlike all the other drugs mentioned so far, it is a tablet that received approval in 2020 exclusively for secondary progressive MS (SPMS).

New treatment options also for relapsing MS (RMS) and relapsing-remitting MS (RRMS):

9.9   Ozanimod and Ponesimod

Ozanimod (Zeposia), which received European marketing authorisation for MS in 2020, and **Ponesimod** (Ponvory), which received marketing authorisation in 2021, are both similar to fingolimod and are taken as a tablet one time daily after a dosing phase.

9.10   Ofatumumab

Ofatumumab (Kesimpta) expanded the therapeutic spectrum in 2021. It belongs to the antibody therapies and is injected subcutaneously once a month after a dosing phase.

9.11   Natalizumab

In 2021, **natalizumab** (Tysabri), which has been approved as an infusion for highly active relapsing-remitting MS since 2006, now also received EU approval in the subcutaneous form. As with the infusion, it is taken at 4-week intervals.

9.12   Diroximel Fumarate

Diroximel fumarate (Vumerity), which also received European marketing authorisation in 2021, concluded the new approvals in 2021. It is a further development of **dimethyl fumarate** (Tecfidera), which has been approved since 2014 and is also taken orally 2 × daily.

As you can see, the MS therapy landscape has developed very rapidly since 2020 and there have never been so many new approvals in MS treatment as in the last 2 years.

9.13   Therapy Goal Today: Individual Therapy—Something for Everyone

As you can see from the medication history, the choice of therapy is increasing, making the treatment of MS more complex, but also more individualised. For whom is which treatment best? For us as treating neurologists, this decision requires a lot of experience and specialised knowledge, because modern MS therapy means a constant examination of new medications and their mechanisms of action, interactions and side effects.

9.13.1 Therapy Concept: Basic and Escalation Therapy

In addition to the constant expansion of the drug therapy landscape, new therapy **concepts** are also being added. For many years, MS therapy was divided into "basic and escalation therapy". **Basic therapy** means the therapy with which treatment is started after diagnosis. As a rule, it is characterised by good tolerability with appropriate efficacy. Substances used in the basic therapy were all interferons, glatiramer acetate, teriflunomide and dimethyl fumarate.

In the case of therapy failure with increasing disease activity, a change was then made to a more effective form of therapy called **escalation therapy.** Drugs used in escalation therapy at the time were natalizumab, fingolimod and alemtuzumab. They are generally characterised by a higher efficacy, but also a greater risk of side effects.

However, the division into basic and escalation therapy corresponds to a very one-dimensional treatment, which presupposes that one always starts "at the base" before escalation can take place. Today, we have moved on from this one-way principle.

9.13.2 New Therapy Concept: Therapy Decisions Based on Prognosis

The principle of basic and escalation therapy has been gradually abandoned in recent years and replaced by the so-called disease-modifying therapy strategy. With this strategy, the therapy decision is more prognosis based. This means that the doctor tries to assess the aggressiveness of the course of the disease from the outset on the basis of certain factors in order to be able to treat it more individually. This approach became possible after some risk factors were identified that are associated with a worse prognosis. Depending on the risk factors present, an individual risk assessment is now carried out before therapy begins and a distinction is made between **"mild/moderate"** and **"active/ highly active"** MS. The appropriate therapy is then selected.

In this way, the therapy concept of "basic/escalation therapy" has become the much more individualised "disease-modifying therapy".

When it is necessary to change therapy as the disease progresses, one no longer speaks of escalation, but of "therapy optimisation".

9.13.3 Prognosis Assessment: There Are Risk Factors

Unfavourable prognostic factors are for example

- Early motor symptoms (i.e. complaints affecting the musculoskeletal system such as paralysis and spasticity)
- A high relapse rate
- Incomplete regression of symptoms after the acute attack
- Early evidence of many T2 lesions in the MRI
- Infratentorial or spinal lesions in the MRI

In addition, risk factors were identified that suggest a more rapid transition to a secondary progressive form of the disease. These appear to include:

- Age at onset
- Relapse frequency
- Time interval between the first two relapses
- Male gender
- Initial degree of disability
- Infratentorial and spinal lesions
- Early T1 hypodense lesions on the MRI

9.13.4 Individual Therapy Decision

If, according to this risk assessment, a mild/moderate course of the disease is to be expected, a "mild/moderate therapy" is chosen, with perhaps somewhat less efficacy, but good tolerability. If a therapy has to be found for a patient with highly active MS, a drug with high efficacy is chosen, whereby a higher risk regarding possible side effects may then have to be accepted.

> Unfortunately, there is (still) no such thing as high effectiveness without corresponding risk, and the effectiveness and risk of the therapy must always be weighed against each other individually.

Substances used to treat the mild/moderate form of progression are all interferons, glatiramer acetate, teriflunomide, dimethyl fumarate and diroximel fumarate. Drugs used to treat the highly active form of progression are nowadays natalizumab, fingolimod, alemtuzumab, cladribine, ocrelizumab, ofatumumab and the new S1P modulators, ozanimod and ponesimod.

The difference to the older concept of basis/escalation therapy is that today, we can treat patients who have a foreseeable higher risk of early disability directly with drugs that were previously reserved for escalation therapy.

> MS therapy has become much more individualised over the years as a result, not only because there are more drugs to choose from, but also because attempts are made to take this individual risk assessment into account when selecting therapy.

The effectiveness on the one hand and the possible side effects and risks on the other must always be weighed up and the benefits and risks considered carefully and individually.

9.13.5 "Hit Hard and Early" and "Treat to Target"

In MS literature, you may come across two other terms: "hit hard and early" and "treat to target". What do they mean? The term "hit hard and early" means an early, highly active therapy to intervene early and aggressively in the autoimmune disease process. Of course, there is a risk of "over-treating". The term "treat to target" (i.e. only treat as far as is necessary), on the other hand, describes a more cautious approach. In this case, the next more intensive therapy is chosen when the therapy fails. This therapy approach may possibly lead to the fact that one or the other person may be under-treated. It is precisely this individual balancing that is complex and difficult in modern MS therapy and requires a lot of experience.

9.13.6 Individual Therapy: Take Life Situation into Account

However, individual therapy does not only mean prognosis-based assessment and weighing of efficacy and risk, but also the consideration of social factors. Thus, one's professional situation, family planning with the desire to have children and comorbidities must be taken into account in order to find the appropriate therapy.

Now that you have become acquainted with the therapy history and the therapy concepts, we will take a closer look at the approved disease-modifying drugs in detail in the next chapter. You will see that a certain basic understanding of the autoimmune process (Chap. 3) helps to understand the specific MS therapies.

10

How the Progression of the Disease Can Be Influenced: The MS Drugs in Detail

As scientific knowledge about the immune system has grown, it has also been possible to better understand the immunological disease mechanisms that make up MS. And from this knowledge, new and increasingly specific drugs have been developed. Thanks to this development, MS can now be treated much better and also more individually, even if the goal of a cure has still not been achieved.

In this chapter, we will take a closer look at the currently approved disease-modifying MS drugs and you will have an overview of the approval criteria, the mechanisms of action, the mode of administration and the frequency of use of the individual drugs.

10.1 The Approved Drugs in Detail

The following disease-modifying drugs or substance groups are currently approved for the treatment of MS, whereby this list is arranged according to the order of their approval

- Interferons: Betaferon/Betaseron, Avonex, Rebif, Extavia, Plegridy
- Glatiramer acetate: Copaxone, Clift
- Natalizumab: Tysabri
- Fingolimod: Gilenya
- Alemtuzumab: Lemtrada
- Teriflunomide: Aubagio

© The Author(s), under exclusive license to Springer-Verlag GmbH, DE, part of Springer Nature 2023
A. Friedrich, *The Multiple Sclerosis Companion*,
https://doi.org/10.1007/978-3-662-67540-3_10

- Dimethyl fumarate: Tecfidera
- Cladribine: Mavenclad
- Ocrelizumab: Ocrevus
- Siponimod: Mayzent
- Ozanimod: Zeposia
- Ofatumumab: Kesimpta
- Ponesimod: Ponvory
- Diroximel fumarate: Vumerity

10.2   How What Works

The mechanisms of action of the drugs are very different, and they attack many different sites in the immune system. The insight you have gained from "A Trip into Our Immune System" (Chap. 3) will now help you to better understand the therapeutic approaches, even though some have not been fully clarified to date.

10.2.1   Interferons and Glatiramer Acetate

Interferons and glatiramer acetate are approved for the "mild/moderate" course of MS. All interferons and glatiramer acetate are approved for relapsing-remitting MS (RRMS), some also for secondary progressive MS (SPMS) and clinically isolated syndrome (CIS). They are injected subcutaneously under the skin; only Avonex is injected into the muscle. Interferons and glatiramer acetate are thought to affect messenger substances in particular by inhibiting the production of pro-inflammatory messengers and promoting the production of anti-inflammatory messengers. They also have a positive effect on regulatory T lymphocytes and an inhibitory one on the inflammation-driving Th1/17 cells. Last but not least, they are also said to influence the permeability of the blood–brain barrier.

10.2.2   Natalizumab

Natalizumab (Tysabri) has been approved for the treatment of highly active relapsing-remitting MS (RRMS) since 2006 and is administered as part of an infusion therapy every 4 weeks. Natalizumab is an antibody that is specifically directed against surface receptors (integrins) on lymphocytes. The inflammatory cells need these receptors to first dock at the blood–brain barrier before they can pass through it. By blocking the surface receptor with natalizumab, the lymphocytes can no longer attach to the vessel wall and therefore can no longer cross the blood–brain barrier. The blood–brain barrier is thus "sealed" against inflammatory cells by natalizumab, so that the lymphocytes can no longer migrate into the CNS.

10.2.3   Fingolimod

Fingolimod (Gilenya) has also been approved since 2011 for the treatment of highly active, relapsing-remitting MS (RRMS) and is taken once daily as a tablet. Fingolimod blocks receptors on the surface of the lymphocytes, the so-called sphingosine-1-phosphate receptors (S1P receptor), which, among other things, mediate the migration of the lymphocytes out of the lymph nodes. In this way, the lymphocytes are "held in the lymph nodes" so that far fewer of them circulate in the blood. This results in the anti-inflammatory effect of fingolimod. With fingolimod, as with natalizumab, there is therefore no destruction of lymphocytes.

10.2.4   Teriflunomide

Teriflunomide (Aubagio) received its approval in 2013 for the mild/moderate course of relapsing-remitting MS (RRMS) and is taken as a tablet once daily. Teriflunomide reversibly (= remediable) inhibits an enzyme in the mitochondria that is needed for the new formation of pyrimidine in the mitochondria. However, the new synthesis of pyrimidine is important for rapidly dividing cells, such as the activated T and B lymphocytes, because pyrimidine is needed as a building material for DNA during cell division. Therefore, the teriflunomide-induced deficiency of the enzyme leads to a reduction in activated lymphocytes.

10.2.5   Dimethyl Fumarate

Dimethyl fumarate (Tecfidera) has also been approved since the beginning of 2014 for the mild/moderate course of relapsing-remitting forms of MS (RRMS). It is taken as a tablet twice a day with a meal. The exact mechanism of action of dimethyl fumarate is not fully understood. Part of the effect is explained by the influence on T-cell differentiation, with promotion of anti-inflammatory Th2 lymphocytes and inhibition of pro-inflammatory Th1 cells. An influence on the antigen-presenting cells as well as an antioxidant effect is assumed.

10.2.6   Alemtuzumab

Alemtuzumab (Lemtrada), approved in 2013 for highly active relapsing-remitting MS (RRMS), was the first MS therapy that did not have to be given continuously. Alemtuzumab is administered as an infusion over 5 days in the first year of therapy and over 3 days in the second year. Alemtuzumab is an antibody that selectively binds to a protein ("CD 52") found in large quantities on the surface of T and B lymphocytes. The antibody binding leads to the destruction ("depletion") of both B and T lymphocytes with a long-lasting effect on the immune system. The idea is that the complete depletion leads to a kind of "reset" with "readjustment" of the immune system with lasting effectiveness. Alemtuzumab is a highly effective therapy but with severe side effects so that today it is more used as a reserve option in highly active MS.

10.2.7   Cladribine

Cladribine (Mavenclad), approved in 2017 for active relapsing MS (RMS), is the first "MS tablet" that does not have to be taken continuously and the only preparation that is prescribed according to weight. As a "short-term oral treatment", cladribine is only taken on a maximum of 10 days within a year over a total treatment period of 2 years. It has a long-lasting and sustainable effect on the immune system. Cladribine is activated in the body itself within the white blood cells. It inhibits DNA synthesis in the B and T lymphocytes as a so-called purine nucleoside analogue, so that the lymphocytes are specifically damaged and die. This leads to a long-lasting reduction in lymphocytes.

10.2.8   Ocrelizumab

Ocrelizumab (Ocrevus) is the first selective B-cell therapy approved for the treatment of MS, i.e. the effect exclusively affects B lymphocytes. Ocrelizumab was approved in 2018 for the treatment of active relapsing MS (RMS) and additionally as the only MS drug so far also for the early **primary progressive** form of MS (PPMS). Ocrelizumab is an antibody. It is selectively directed against a surface protein ("CD20") that is only found on B lymphocytes.

After ocrelizumab binds to the CD20 surface protein of the B cells, these B lymphocytes are rapidly destroyed. However, since the CD20 proteins are not present on the stem cells nor on the plasma cells, the ability to form new cells and the immunological long-term memory are largely preserved. Ocrelizumab is administered semi-annually as an infusion therapy.

And now, what else has been added since 2020 when this book was first published in German.

10.2.9   Siponimod

Siponimod (Mayzent) entered the European market in 2020 and is the first and so far only drug approved exclusively for the treatment of secondary progressive MS (SPMS). The prerequisite for siponimod treatment in SPMS is that the disease has still shown some activity in the form of clinical relapses or inflammatory MRI activity in the last 2 years. Siponimod is a selective sphingosine-1-phosphate (S1P) receptor modulator that prevents lymphocytes from migrating out of lymph nodes (similar to fingolimod). Siponimod is taken in tablet form once a day after a 5-day build-up phase. Since there are a few people who metabolise the drug poorly or not at all, the so-called metabolisation status must be checked by a blood or saliva test before the first dose is taken in order to determine the appropriate siponimod dose.

10.2.10   Ozanimod

Ozanimod (Zeposia) was approved in the EU in 2020 for the treatment of adult MS patients with active relapsing-remitting MS (RRMS).

It is as fingolimod (Gilenya), a selective S1P receptor modulator that is also taken orally and prevents lymphocytes from migrating out of the lymph nodes. Zeposia also needs to be slowly dosed up or increased, over 7 days using a starter pack, before reaching the maintenance dose of one tablet daily from day 8. It has shown to have fewer side effects, especially cardiovascular side effects, than fingolimod.

Zeposia has since received a marketing authorisation extension in 2022 and is now also used in addition to MS, in moderate and severe active ulcerative colitis, a chronic inflammatory disease of the colon.

10.2.11 Ofatumumab

Ofatumumab (Kesimpta), like ocrelizumab (Ocrevus), is another anti-CD20 antibody that targets the surface proteins ("CD20") of B lymphocytes and destroys them after binding.

Approved in 2021 for the treatment of active relapsing MS in adults (RMS), it is injected subcutaneously.

After a 1-month dosing phase, it is subsequently applied subcutaneously once a month. Ofatumumab is the first B-cell-depleting agent that can be injected independently by the patient at home after therapy adjustment under guidance.

10.2.12 Natalizumab Subcutaneous (s.c.)

In 2021, natalizumab (Tysabri), which has been approved since 2006, received EU approval for subcutaneous administration, whereas previously it could only be given as infusion therapy. Like intravenous Tysabri, the subcutaneous version is approved for the treatment of highly active relapsing-remitting MS (RRMS).

The injections in the form of two pre-filled syringes are both administered subcutaneously by healthcare professionals at 4-week intervals. At least for the first six injections, as with the infusion, a 1-hour follow-up period is necessary. This may be omitted from the seventh injection onwards at the discretion of the practitioner.

10.2.13 Ponesimod

Ponesimod (Ponvory), like ozanimod, is an oral selective S1P receptor modulator that is slowly administered over 14 days according to a fixed-dose titration schedule. From day 15, the maintenance dose is reached and taken once in the morning in the form of one tablet. Ponesimod received European marketing authorisation in 2021 for the treatment of adult patients with active relapsing MS (RMS).

10.2.14 Diroximel Fumarate

Diroximel fumarate (Vumerity) received European marketing authorisation in 2021 for the treatment of adults with relapsing-remitting MS (RRMS).

Diroximel fumarate is a further development of dimethyl fumarate (Tecfidera), which has already been approved since 2014 and has better gastrointestinal tolerability. It is taken twice daily in the form of two tablets in the morning and two tablets in the evening.

10.3 No Effect Without Side Effect

As you have read, all of the MS drugs presented here influence the immune system in different ways, whose task it is to keep infections and also degenerative cells in check or to fight them off. This explains some side effects, especially with the drugs that are used to treat highly active MS. The most important of these is an **increased tendency to infection**, which is reported as a side effect in different ways with all highly active MS drugs. For this reason, active infections must be ruled out by blood tests before starting therapy with these drugs. If infections were present and the immune system was "throttled", the responsible viruses/bacteria would have an easy time and the infectious disease could worsen. In addition, before starting therapy, the vaccination status is checked and the vaccination record is updated if necessary. All recommended vaccinations should be refreshed before starting therapy (Chap. 12: "MS and Vaccination"). In addition, pregnancy must be safely ruled out before starting therapy (Chap. 13)!

10.4 JCV and PML: What Is It?

A particular example of a rare but very serious infection during therapy is **progressive multifocal leukoencephalopathy (PML).** This extremely rare disease is a viral infection with the **John Cunningham virus (JCV)** or JC virus for short. The virus is named after the patient in whom it was first discovered in 1971. It is widespread and is probably acquired in childhood. The JC virus lies dormant in the body of many people (>70%) and is easily kept in check by a healthy immune system. However, if the immune system is weakened by a severe immune deficiency (e.g. AIDS), the dormant virus can be reactivated, i.e. awakened. It then spreads through the body and once in the CNS, these viruses attack the oligodendrocytes and destroy them. The oligodendrocytes are the myelin producers that you learned about in Chap. 3. If these myelin producers are destroyed, there is increasing demyelination of the central nervous system, but this time not—as in MS—through a local autoimmune attack, but through the increasing viral attack. The symptoms depend on the location of the damage and lead to the corresponding neuro-logical deficits of PML, which can initially be very similar to an MS relapse. Unlike the relapse, however, the symptoms do not subside again, but rather the neurological deficits become progressively worse as the virus spreads. PML disease leads to death if it is not recognised in time.

So much for JCV and PML—but what does this have to do with MS therapy? The very rare PML disease was observed more frequently during therapy with natalizumab (Tysabri), especially after many years of treatment. In the meantime, however, isolated cases of PML have also been observed during therapy with fingolimod (Gilenya), dimethyl fumarate (Tecfidera) and also ocrelizumab (Ocrevus). Theoretically, any drug that strongly influences the immune system can trigger PML, but this is extremely rare.

It is now well known which patients have an increased risk of developing PML. This risk group primarily includes patients who are proven JC virus carriers and have been treated with natalizumab for more than 2 years. Fortunately, there is now the possibility of measuring a JCV antibody titre (JCV antibody index), which is related to the risk of PML in JCV-positive patients (i.e. virus carriers). The risk of a possible infection can now be assessed much better. The JCV virus status is therefore checked before a therapy deci-sion is made and is also checked regularly during natalizumab therapy.

If PML is suspected, a lumbar puncture is performed (Chap. 5) and the virus can then be detected in the laboratory via its DNA. In addition, typical changes show up in the MRI, so that an MRI must be performed quickly in every suspected case.

You can see from this example that risk and benefit cannot always be sepa-rated. Highly effective therapies, which become necessary when there is a threat of rapidly increasing disability due to MS, must always be weighed against the possible risks. Through increasing knowledge about our immune system and increasing experience with the highly active drugs, the risks are becoming more and more calculable, but they still need to be weighed up conscientiously before starting therapy.

10.5   Regulatory Studies, Expert Information and "Real-World Data"

As you have seen from the long list of MS drugs, the drugs differ in terms of their approval, mechanism of action, mode of administration and frequency of use. They also differ in their individual side effect profile and therapy monitoring. Drug-specific side effects and different therapy monitoring are not discussed in detail in this companion, as this would require a very detailed presentation. For this purpose, I would like to refer to the approval studies as well as to the corresponding technical information of the respective medicines, which is constantly updated, especially for newer preparations.

When evaluating the results of approval studies, you should always take into account that studies with a limited number of patients are conducted for a limited observation period with a clearly defined patient clientele. Therefore, it is important to closely observe the effect and side effect of every newly approved drug, especially after its approval, under real everyday conditions, which is then called "real-world data". If side effects occur, they should be reported immediately.

And something else is worth mentioning when assessing study results—they cannot be compared. Each study is conducted under different conditions with non-comparable patient populations. A true comparison of drugs is therefore only possible through **direct** comparative studies, so-called "head-to-head" studies. These are clinical trials in which one active substance is compared directly against another active substance under controlled conditions. However, such "head-to-head" studies rarely exist.

Now that you know which medicines are available for which indications and with what effect, the question arises in the course of therapy: How can I tell if my therapy is working? How can therapy success be measured? We will explore these questions in the next chapter, "The Therapy Goal Has a Name: NEDA".

11

The Therapy Goal Has a Name: NEDA

How do we monitor a therapy, i.e. how do we determine whether the therapy we have started is really effective? Today, we have high expectations for a successful MS therapy. Because if we cannot cure MS so far, we at least want to stop the progression of the disease.

> This therapeutic goal is called "NEDA" and stands for "no evidence of disease activity".

To achieve the desired therapy goal, namely "complete freedom from clinical and paraclinical disease activity", three parameters are observed during therapy ("NEDA 3"). These three parameters are the **relapse activity** and the so-called **disability progression** for the "clinical disease activity", as well as the **MRI progression** for the "paraclinical disease activity" (in medicine, paraclinical is the term used for examination results that can be determined by technical means—for example, blood examination in the laboratory or imaging of the body with radiological equipment). Let us start with the paraclinical disease activity.

11.1 Paraclinical Course Parameters: MRI

The MRI as a paraclinical parameter for monitoring the course of therapy is of great importance in therapy monitoring because it can detect a possible "silent" progression of the disease (i.e. without noticeable symptoms). In the

A. Friedrich, *The Multiple Sclerosis Companion*, https://doi.org/10.1007/978-3-662-67540-3_11

MRI, attention is paid to new and/or enlarging inflammatory lesions compared to pre-MRI.

> If new or enlarging lesions are detected in the MRI, this is a sign of disease progression and thus the therapeutic goal of NEDA would not be achieved (▶ Sect. 4.8).

11.2 Dreams of the Future: Neurofilaments

In addition to the MRI, other paraclinical markers would be desired that could be used to read the course of the disease and possible progression at an early stage. The so-called neurofilaments are currently in focus here. The detection of neurofilaments (NFLs) in cerebrospinal fluid and now also in serum could possibly become such a biomarker in the future. Neurofilaments are proteins that are released when nerve cells die. However, they are not MS specific. They provide an indication of neuronal damage and are seen as a prognostic biomarker of neuronal cell death. Whether they can be routinely used in monitoring the course of MS therapy has not yet been conclusively clarified.

11.3 Clinical Course Parameters: Relapse Rate and Disability Progression

In addition to the MRI, two clinical parameters (i.e. parameters that become noticeable through symptoms) are used to monitor the course of therapy, namely relapse activity and disability progression, which are recorded through regular neurological check-ups.

> If relapses or clinical deterioration in the neurological examination occur during therapy, resulting in increasing disability, this indicates the progression of the disease. This would mean that the NEDA therapy goal has not been achieved.

While a relapse is easily recognisable as an acute event, a slowly progressing deterioration of the disabilities caused by MS (disability progression) is often much more difficult to detect over the course of time because it usually happens insidiously.

11.4   The EDSS Score Shows Disability Progression

The "EDSS score" (expanded disability status scale), a scale that provides information about the degree of disability of an MS patient, is used to better record and understand the gradual progression of the disease over time. This scale is based on the standardised neurological examination, in which seven different neurological functional systems (FS) are tested. These functional systems tested include vision, motor function, brainstem function, coordination, sensitivity, bladder and bowel function and brain performance.

An EDSS of 0 means no neurological abnormalities, an EDSS of 9 corresponds to bedriddenness and an EDSS of 10 means death by MS (● Fig 11.1).

> A deterioration in the EDSS score over time indicates progression of the disease. This means that the therapy goal NEDA would not be achieved.

If you take a close look at the scale, you will notice that the ability to walk is particularly important in the EDSS scale. While a score of 3 still means unrestricted walking ability without assistance, from an EDSS of 4, the score is predominantly determined by the walking ability. With a score of 4, the person concerned is still able to walk at least 500 m without assistance; with a score of 5, at least 200 m is possible; with a score of 6, a walking aid is needed to walk 100 m; with 7, the ability to walk with assistance is only possible for a maximum of 5 m; 8 means constantly dependent on a wheelchair; and 9 indicates bedriddenness.

The EDSS score is criticised for taking much less account of non-motor symptoms such as chronic fatigue syndrome and limitations in cognition (concentration, comprehension, memory), even though these symptoms can be even more burdensome for some people than the limited walking distance.

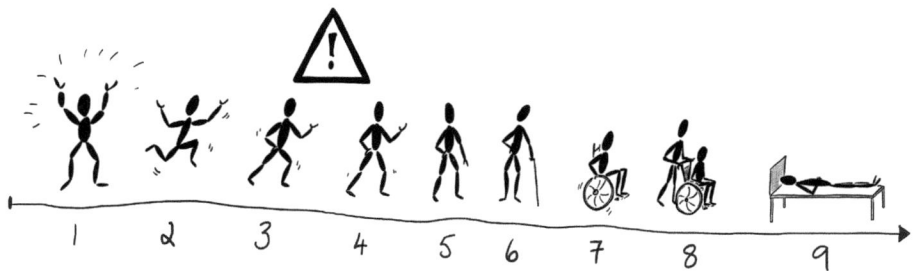

Fig. 11.1 Assessment of disability: EDSS score

11.5   The Hidden Symptoms: Fatigue and Cognition

The non-motor symptoms such as the limitations in cognitive performance or constant tiredness (fatigue) have not been given sufficient attention for a long time. However, studies show that more than 70% of MS patients suffer from these hidden symptoms during the course of the disease.

Standardised neuropsychological tests have shown that cognitive changes typical of MS are particularly evident in the slowing down of information processing (so-called information processing speed). In addition, concentration problems and restrictions in sustained attention are typical. Also, the so-called mental flexibility with loss of multitasking (i.e. the ability to keep several tasks in mind at the same time) can also be impaired.

Furthermore, MS can lead to a pronounced fatigue syndrome. This syndrome describes an abnormal physical and cognitive fatigability, lack of energy and exhaustion, which is often described by those affected "as if the plug had been pulled". There are some patients who even name this symptom as their worst complaint.

Symptoms such as fatigue syndrome and/or limitations in cognitive performance have a significant impact on social life and professional activity, so that some affected persons are more restricted in their everyday working life than by physical complaints. Therefore, it is important to take these changes into account in the course of the disease. Unfortunately, there are still no effective therapies for either cognitive changes or fatigue syndrome. However, there are indications in the literature that moderate endurance and brain power training have a positive effect on cognitive performance. I would also like to refer to the influence of nutrition on fatigue symptoms in this context (▶ Part III).

11.6   In a Nutshell

In everyday clinical practice, the three parameters of MRI progression, relapse frequency and disability progression are regularly checked for therapy monitoring ("NEDA-3"). As monitoring of the therapy goal, the parameters cognition ("NEDA-4") and brain atrophy ("NEDA-5") are also recorded, especially in the context of studies. Achieving the therapy goal NEDA is the wishful thinking of every modern MS therapy. If it is not achieved, a change in therapy should be considered at an early stage to avoid further progression of the disease.

12

MS and Vaccinations

Protective vaccinations protect against infectious diseases that can be potentially life-threatening, making vaccinations one of the most effective preventive measures in medicine. How important it is to have an effective vaccine at hand against diseases is something we—in corona times—have experienced first-hand.

12.1 Active and Passive Vaccination

In principle, a distinction is made in vaccinations between so-called active and passive vaccines. In the case of "**active vaccination**", the body must actively do something, because either attenuated pathogens (live vaccines) or dead components of these pathogens (inactivated vaccines) are administered to the body in small doses as a vaccine. Against these pathogens or their components, the body then forms "specially made antibodies" and also memory cells, as described in Chap. 3. Do you remember the "reminder function"? If a vaccinated person is later infected with the real pathogen, this function takes effect and memory cells are activated. This very quickly leads to effective antibody formation and defence reaction against the invader whose mugshot was already listed in the pathogen file of the immune system due to the vaccination.

The situation is completely different with the so-called "**passive vaccination**". Here, the body does not need to do anything on its own, because ready-made, pathogen-specific antibodies from another person who has

A. Friedrich, *The Multiple Sclerosis Companion*,
https://doi.org/10.1007/978-3-662-67540-3_12

already acquired immunity against this invader are administered. The foreign antibodies then fight the enemy and eliminate it. However, no immunity is gained in this process.

> Active vaccinations serve as a preventive measure and are divided into inactivated and live vaccinations. In the case of vaccinations with an inactivated vaccine, the pathogens are dead; in the case of vaccinations with a live vaccine, on the other hand, the pathogens are attenuated but still potentially capable of reproducing.

You can now easily imagine that MS patients and immunocompromised people should not be given live vaccines; at least this must be considered very carefully in each individual case, taking into account the risk-benefit ratio. In contrast, inactivated vaccines can also be administered to immunocompromised people without any problems.

12.2   Why Is the Vaccination Issue So Important in MS Now?

The vaccination issue is very important because the necessary therapies (such as cortisone therapy in acute relapses and the course-modifying drugs) suppress the immune system to varying degrees. On the one hand, this is exactly the purpose of MS therapy, but on the other hand, it is often associated with an increased risk of infection, as you have already learned in Chap. 10. To minimise this risk, it is important to update one's vaccination protection, especially before starting treatment for highly active MS. This is a preventive measure. Updating one's vaccination certificate is therefore recommended for every MS patient at an early stage and is even required before starting therapy with drugs such as alemtuzumab, ocrelizumab, ofatumumab, fingolimod, ozanimod, ponesimod, siponimod and cladribine.

In Germany, where I live, the Permanent Vaccination Commission (STIKO) at the Robert Koch Institute (RKI) regularly issues vaccination recommendations. In addition to the usual vaccinations, the STIKO also explicitly recommends the flu vaccination for MS patients. You can also read these recommendations on the internet at www.rki.de. Please check with the relevant vaccination commission or authorities in the country in which you live.

> Ideally, all vaccinations recommended should be carried out and completed before the start of therapy. The vaccinations should be carried out during a stable phase of the disease, i.e. not in an acute episode and not during cortisone therapy.

12.3 Distance Good: All Good

It is recommended to keep an interval of at least 4–6 weeks between a relapse with cortisone treatment and a vaccination. Depending on the treatment, different intervals (usually 4–6 weeks) must also be observed between a vaccination and the start of a highly active MS therapy in order to achieve maximum vaccination success. Since the success of the vaccination, as described above, depends on the formation of antibodies, which in turn are formed by the plasma cells (which come from the B lymphocytes), you can imagine that under a B-cell-destroying therapy, such as with ocrelizumab, ofatumumab and alemtuzumab, sufficient vaccination success fails to materialise. This is why it is so important to vaccinate before starting therapy.

- Examples of inactivated vaccinations: influenza, pneumococci, meningococci, hepatitis B, herpes zoster, human papillomavirus (HPV) and TBE (early summer meningoencephalitis).
- Examples of live vaccinations: measles, mumps, rubella, varicella zoster (= chickenpox).

After this chapter, "MS and Vaccinations", we will look at another special topic in the following, namely family planning in the chapter "MS and the Desire to Have Children".

13

MS and the Desire to Have Children

Of course, patients with MS can get pregnant! The fertility of women and men with MS is not limited.

> The pregnancy of a woman with MS is not a high-risk pregnancy!

The pregnancy courses of women with MS and women without MS do not differ from each other. Furthermore, a negative effect neither on the child's development nor on the birth could be determined. Even childbirth itself does not involve any greater risk than that in women not affected by MS. There are also no objections to spinal or peridural anaesthesia (PDA) during delivery.

Pregnancy itself even has a certain protective effect for the woman affected by MS, because the relapse rate tends to decrease during pregnancy. However, since statistically there is an increase in the relapse rate in the first 3 months after delivery, this phase should be planned early on.

> The recommended course of action after delivery depends on the disease activity that existed before pregnancy.

For patients to receive individual and correct advice **before** they become pregnant, it is essential that they let their neurologist know about their family planning, because different rules apply depending on which medication they are taking.

A. Friedrich, *The Multiple Sclerosis Companion*,
https://doi.org/10.1007/978-3-662-67540-3_13

Effective contraception is necessary under almost all course-modifying MS therapies. There has been an exception to this since October 2019, as interferon-beta may, if clinically necessary, also be continued during pregnancy in RRMS, and the same applies to glatiramer acetate, subject to a risk/benefit assessment.

13.1   The Importance of Pregnancy Registers and MS

Many of the findings described above come from pregnancy registers.

In Germany, there is the German Multiple Sclerosis and Fertility Registry (DMSKW). In the UK, there is the UK MS Pregnancy Register. The DMSKW has existed since 2002 and is run in Bochum as a German-speaking MS and fertility registry. The DMSKW is an independent initiative that collects data and experience values on pregnancies or fertility treatments of MS patients.

The UK MS Pregnancy Register is also a patient-facing register, so people with MS can sign up directly without needing to go through their neurologist. The only real criteria are that they have MS and are pregnant. It collects information on things like DMT exposure, supplement use, breastfeeding and mood disorders in pregnancy.

This data is increasingly being used to gain knowledge about pregnancy in MS, which can be passed on as recommendations to people with MS.

In this respect, I would like to motivate everyone to contact the corresponding addresses (see below), if they are planning a pregnancy or if a pregnancy has already occurred.

You can also get a lot of important information there about breastfeeding, because there is no reason not to breastfeed if you have MS. If the patient decides against breastfeeding, a quick resumption of MS therapy after delivery is usually recommended.

- For detailed information on the topic of MS and the desire to have children, I refer you to the following addresses:
  Professor Dr. med. Kerstin Hellwig, Neurological Clinic, St Josef Hospital Bochum.
      www.ms-und-kinderwunsch.de
  Kerstin.Hellwig@ruhr-uni-bochum.de
  Dr. Ruth Dobson, Queen Mary University London
  www.ukmsregister.org/pregnancy
  mspregnancy@ukmsregister.org

13.2   MS Is Not a Hereditary Disease

Of course, there is a fear among MS sufferers with pregnancy planning that MS may be inherited. However, it is known from studies on twins and family studies that genetic factors do play a role, but only a subordinate one. MS is not a "hereditary disease". Let us first look at the risk of developing MS in the general population: It is 0.1–0.2% and increases to 2% if one parent has the disease. Although 2% might sound like a lot at first, if we look at this risk the other way round, there is a 98% chance that the child will not develop MS. If both parents have MS, the risk increases to 20%. So, there is a dependency on the degree of relationship.

Studies on twins have shown that if an identical twin suffers from MS, the risk of the other twin also suffering from MS is not 100%, but only 25–30%, even though they have exactly the same genetic make-up. Conversely, this means that genetics is not everything, because the rest, namely the remaining 70–75%, is attributed to environmental influences, which are thus to be rated much higher than the genetic component.

> It is likely that a genetic predisposition to the disease (susceptibility) is inherited, which can be modified by environmental factors.

For this reason, Part III of the book, which now follows, is particularly close to my heart, as in this part we will take a closer look at environmental factors and ask: "What can I do myself?"

Part III

MS: And What You Can Do Yourself

14

Self-Initiative Helps

The good news is: Yes, everyone affected can do a lot themselves! To start with, I would like to tell you a short story of my own. A few years ago, I went through a phase where I increasingly lacked drive, was constantly tired and had trouble concentrating; my joints and muscles hurt especially in the morning; and my mood was not the best either. Everyday things in life that otherwise went easily became more difficult and sluggish. At that time, I read a report about the success of vegetarian and vegan diets for such issues, so I decided to try it out for myself. Together, we changed our diet at home to a vegetarian, i.e. plant-based diet. We also reduced sugar and wheat products. About 4 weeks later, we both noticed that we felt more alert and fresh. My daytime fatigue and lack of concentration disappeared, my drive returned to normal and even my joint and muscle pain subsided. I felt fit and efficient again.

14.1 From Self-Experimentation to Case Reports

I passed on this very interesting personal experience to patients who complained of severe fatigue. Since MS patients often suffer from chronic fatigue syndrome (Chap. 13), for which orthodox medicine has no therapeutic answer so far, it made sense to tell them about my own experiences through dietary changes. And lo and behold, many who consistently changed their diet had comparable experiences. They also reported a clear improvement in fatigue with an increase in performance. Some even experienced a complete

A. Friedrich, *The Multiple Sclerosis Companion*, https://doi.org/10.1007/978-3-662-67540-3_14

regression of fatigue symptoms, such as in the case of a 21-year-old patient E. whom I would like to introduce briefly here.

E. was diagnosed with MS after a visual disturbance occurred, and many MS-typical lesions were found in the MRI of the skull. Unfortunately, these were located in prognostically unfavourable places in the brainstem, in the cerebellum and at several levels of the spinal cord. MS-typical changes were also found in the cerebrospinal fluid. After clarifying the diagnosis, we started immunomodulatory therapy immediately. During the course of treatment, however, the patient had a new relapse with sensory disturbances in the arms and legs, and the MRI control showed a clear deterioration with fresh contrast-enhancing lesions. Although the relapse symptoms completely disappeared after cortisone therapy, a very stressful and persistent fatigue set in, which severely impaired the young woman's daily activities. She had to lie down regularly during the day just to cope with the demands of everyday life. Due to the clinical deterioration and MRI progression, we changed the MS therapy. However, because my patient continued to complain about the performance-limiting fatigue, I told her about my positive experience with dietary changes. I recommended a plant-based, fibre-rich whole-food diet with lots of green vegetables, pulses, nuts, omega-3-rich oils and as far as possible no sugar or wheat products. In the broadest sense, this dietary recommendation can be summarised briefly as a vegetarian diet with some fish or even a Mediterranean diet without meat. What happened to E. just afterwards was remarkable. The fatigue disappeared in the young woman, her drive returned, she became efficient again and the regular afternoon naps were no longer necessary. As an additional positive side effect, the overweight young woman slowly but steadily lost a total of 20 kg in weight within 2 years and is now of normal weight. The patient has been free of relapses since then, has a stable EDSS and the MRI checks, which have been carried out regularly for years, have not shown any new lesions to date. She feels better than ever, and E. is not an isolated case.

Another patient A. suffered from neurodermatitis in addition to MS with pronounced fatigue syndrome. After the recommended change in diet, she reported enthusiastically that not only the fatigue symptoms but also the skin changes had disappeared. After a "Christmas diet slip" with lots of animal fats, sugar and wheat products, both the fatigue and the neurodermitic skin changes reappeared. However, they completely disappeared again after she had resumed her tried and tested nutritional concept.

Though these patient reports remain individual case descriptions, they are not proof. And of course, both patients continued the recommended immunomodulatory therapy in addition to the dietary changes, but this alone had no positive effect on the fatigue syndrome in these two patients.

14.2   The Intestine in the Focus of Research

Inspired by these positive practical experiences, I began to research what could be found in the literature on nutrition, immune system and autoimmune diseases and whether there might be a scientific justification for the optimistic observations from everyday practice. I have found many interesting observations, studies and animal experiments on the influence of nutrition on the intestine, its bacterial colonisation and the possible consequences for the immune system and have compiled them for you here. The gut and the gut-brain axis are increasingly the focus of research.

Therefore, we will have a closer look at these connections in the following pages. There is much to suggest that we are only at the beginning of a new discovery, and that we will hear much more in the future about the connections between nutrition, intestinal colonisation, immune system and brain. Since neurologists have been less familiar with the gut and gastroenterologists are not specialists in the nervous system, we may have to work together more across the disciplines again, because nothing in the body happens in isolation.

15

Forest Fire MS

Let us imagine a forest fire. It is put out and extinguished, and it seems successful at first. But again and again, someone ignites and starts new small fires, which in turn spread needing to be extinguished again. Does it make sense to extinguish the forest fire? Of course, you say, of course it makes sense to extinguish the forest fire. Does it make sense to identify the "igniters"? Of course, right?

Are there perhaps "igniters" in MS? Are there factors that perhaps "ignite" again and again and keep rekindling the forest fire in the most diverse places? Do we extinguish the "small new fires" with cortisone but have not yet been able to identify and eliminate the igniters?

15.1 The MS Numbers Are Increasing

The number of people with MS is steadily increasing and has approximately doubled in the last 40 years. In Germany, the number is now over 240,000. In the UK, it is approximately 130,000, and in Europe, it is estimated that nearly 1 million people are affected; worldwide, the figure is about 2.5 million. On the one hand, there are more and more MS therapies available, and on the other hand, there are more and more new cases. Are we only attacking one side with our current MS treatment?

Studies by the World Health Organization (WHO) show a particularly high incidence of MS worldwide in Europe and North America and, interestingly, especially in the high-income groups of the various countries. There are

A. Friedrich, *The Multiple Sclerosis Companion*, https://doi.org/10.1007/978-3-662-67540-3_15

indications that MS occurs mainly in countries with a higher gross national product and thus greater purchasing power. Is MS a "disease of affluence" like many other diseases? Are there causative lifestyle factors that "ignite" it?

Many studies deal with this question, because it is not only MS that has increased considerably in the last decades. Even among young people, the number of diabetes sufferers has risen drastically, as has the number of overweight people and the number of people with high blood pressure. Cardiovascular diseases are becoming more frequent, as are new cancers, especially breast, prostate and colon carcinomas.

15.2   Not Victims of Our Genes: Environmental Factors in Our Sights

We know from studies on twins that only about 30% of the risk of disease is genetic; the rest—and thus 70%—is determined by environmental factors. This means that genetics obviously only plays a subordinate role, and the good news is therefore:

> We are not victims of our genes!

There are now many studies that have identified individual environmental influences as possible risk factors for MS. As far as is known, these include obesity, nicotine, high salt consumption, stress, lack of sunlight and vitamin D deficiency. Several studies have shown that overweight young women are three times more likely to develop MS than those of normal weight. Smoking leads to a 1.5-fold increase in risk. It not only influences the progression of the disease, but also accelerates the transition from the relapsing-remitting form (RRMS) to the secondary progressive form of MS (SPMS). High salt consumption, which is widespread in the Western world, is also discussed as a risk factor in the development of autoimmune diseases, because salt can activate inflammatory Th17 cells and pro-inflammatory messenger substances. Sunlight and vitamin D, on the other hand, seem to have an anti-inflammatory effect on the immune system (Chap. 24, Vitamin D).

Recent studies have focused on the connection between nutrition and immune system. In particular, the influence of various fats on the intestine and the immune system, especially, long-chain fatty acids and so-called transfats, is said to have unfavourable effects, while other fats have a very positive effect on health—because fat is not just fat. If environmental factors play a role in the risk of disease and the course of MS, it seems sensible to identify these possibly "igniting" environmental factors and examine them more closely. In the following chapters, we will have a closer look at these environmental factors because they are important when it comes to answering the question: What can I do myself?

16

Western Diet and Blue Zones

When we think about environmental factors, we can ask ourselves what has actually changed in the last few decades (Fig. 16.1). The answer is:

Nothing has changed so massively in the industrial nations as **our diet!**

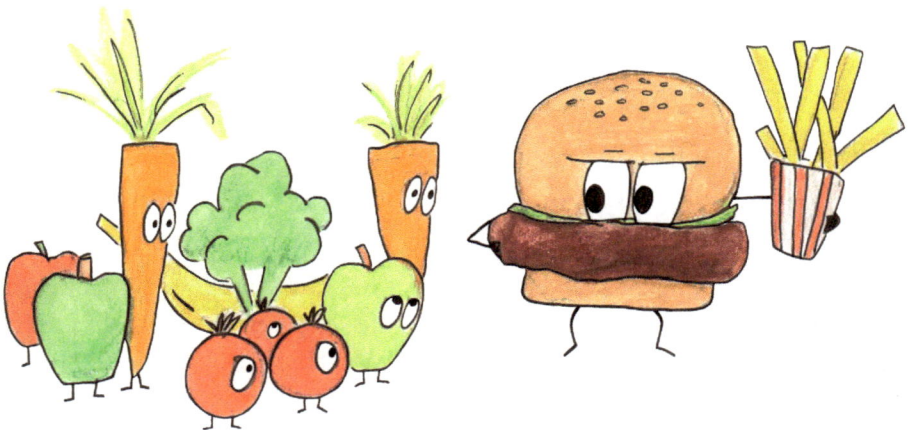

Fig. 16.1 Nutrition yesterday and today

What was a predominantly plant-based, high-fibre diet with vegetable fats, vegetable proteins, secondary plant substances through lots of vegetables, mushrooms, spices, herbs, nuts and little meat has today become a diet that consists mainly of animal fats and animal proteins. In addition, there is a high proportion of sugar and salt as well as industrially produced fats that the body did not know before.

16.1   Our Diet Has Changed: "Western Diet"

Today's so-called "Western diet" is characterised by convenience foods with often high hidden sugar and salt content, hydrogenated fats, preservatives, emulsifiers and flavour enhancers, in short: many unhealthy and/or chemical ingredients. Vegetables or salad leaves often appear only for decorative purposes. In addition, there is a high level of stress, possibly coupled with regular alcohol and nicotine consumption. The hectic pace and lack of time in everyday life often prevent us from buying fresh ingredients and preparing them ourselves.

> Heating up ready-made products is quicker and more practical in today's hectic world. And that is where the problem begins, because ready-made products often contain a lot of things we would not have suspected and are often not good for the body.

16.2   Ready-Made Products: Chemistry Replaces Nature

We live in a time when a strawberry yoghurt has not come into contact with a single strawberry. Chemistry replaces nature, and very often with a high sugar content. The WHO recommends no more than a daily amount of 25 g of added sugar for women and 36 g for men. Across Europe, the UK and the USA, and much of the world, the number consumed is nearly four or five times the recommended amount.

For example, every German now consumes an average of about 31 kg of household sugar per year, which is about 86 g per day or the equivalent of **29 sugar cubes per day,** because one cube contains 3 g of sugar. A large amount of this hidden sugar is consumed today through soft drinks. But even if you think you do not actually eat much sweet stuff, you will be surprised because you can find out how much sugar you are consuming from the nutritional value table on the packaging label. You will find out, for example, that a 400 g package of white cabbage salad contains 56 g of sugar (= 18.7 sugar cubes) and the Pizza Hawaii also contains 22 g, i.e. 7 sugar cubes. Would you have thought that? But not only the hidden sugars are a problem.

An equally important issue is the high proportion of hidden, artificially hydrogenated, vegetable fats in our "Western diet". Hardened vegetable fats are produced industrially. The vegetable fats, which are liquid under normal circumstances, are heated strongly and harden in the process. Because these hardened fats have a longer shelf life, they are often used in ready-made products, such as chocolate bars, spreads, margarine, baked goods and many other industrially manufactured products. These hydrogenated vegetable fats are declared as "vegetable fats" on the packaging, and the consumer thinks, because they are "vegetable", that it is something good for the body. Unfortunately, the opposite is the case. A particularly harmful fat among the fats is not even mentioned in the nutritional value table of the packaging, the so-called trans-fats which are associated with a high risk of coronary heart disease. Trans-fats are unnatural, new fats that are an unwanted by-product of the industrial hardening process of vegetable fats. Trans-fats are present in hardened vegetable fats in varying percentages and are found, for example, in margarine, French fries, crisps and other fried products. There are clear indications that trans-fats are, to a large extent, responsible for fuelling inflammatory processes and for the development of vascular calcification and thus for strokes and heart attacks.

So not all fats are the same! And there is a huge difference between consuming these artificially hydrogenated vegetable fats and trans-fats and consuming large amounts of linseed or olive oil. Because, as you will see in the studies in this chapter, there is evidence that with olive oil, an important ingredient of the Mediterranean diet, you can even significantly reduce the risk of heart attacks, strokes and cancer.

> The choice of fats is therefore of immense importance for our health.

16.3   Create Awareness

I am not writing this to spoil your appetite, but merely to raise awareness of what we often, perhaps unknowingly, ingest every day with our "Western diet".

> What we take in, what we "nourish" our body with, has a direct influence on our health!

Even the Greek physician and father of medicine, Hippocrates of Kos (460 to 377 BC), said: "Let your food be your medicine and your medicine be your food".

16.4 "Blue Zones": Healthy Ageing

Have you ever heard about "Blue Zones"? There are areas where people are much less likely to live with chronic illnesses and who grow particularly old and often remain mentally alert and physically healthy into old age. These regions are called "Blue Zones". The Blue Zones have the world's highest density of over 100-year-olds—healthy 100-year-olds! The term "Blue Zones" comes from the American author Dan Buettner, who led a National Geographic expedition. He investigated this phenomenon with an expert team of anthropologists, historians, nutritionists and geneticists and published the results for National Geographic under the title "The Secrets of a Long Life". The five zones discovered by Dan Buettner are located in Okinawa (Japan), Ikaria (Greece), Sardinia (Italy), Loma Linda (Southern California) and the Nicoya Peninsula (Costa Rica).

The interesting thing about the Blue Zones is that they are all characterised by a special diet that is very different from our "Western diet". The meals are freshly prepared, predominantly plant based and high in fibre and contain many good oils. Seasonal foods are used, most of which come from the region. Meat and milk are rarely consumed, and thus little animal fat and protein are consumed.

Traditional cuisine in Okinawa favours lots of tofu, seaweed, fish, soybean oil, brown rice, green tea and bitter melons. In Ikaria and Sardinia, the Mediterranean diet consists mainly of vegetables, fruit, nuts, herbs and spices, cold-pressed olive oil, rapeseed oil and avocados, while in Costa Rica, the diet is also plant based and high in fibre, with beans. Soft drinks and sugary drinks are virtually unknown in these regions.

Of the five Blue Zones places, Loma Linda, a town in Southern California, is probably particularly surprising. In Loma Linda, people belong to the Seventh-day Adventist Church, a Protestant religious community. The members of this religious community eat a vegetarian diet. They abstain from nicotine and alcohol, and physical activity is a regular part of their daily programme.

It is interesting that people from the Blue Zones are not only getting older, but the diseases found in countries where a Western diet is consumed such as diabetes, cardiovascular diseases, dementia or cancer are much less common in the Blue Zones.

Of course, these findings are only observations and not yet proof. However, there are now many studies on the links between lifestyle, diet and chronic diseases, ranging from studies with very small numbers of cases to huge, epidemiological studies such as "The China Study". What they all have in common is the evidence for a clear link between plant-based nutrition and health.

17

Nutrition Works

What is it about plant based and high fibre? And what actually are dietary fibres? Dietary fibres are food components that are indigestible for the human body (i.e. supposed "fibre" that cannot be utilised), mostly from carbohydrates. They are predominantly found in plant foods and are contained, for example, in vegetables, fruits, cereals, pulses, nuts and wholemeal products.

17.1 Dietary Fibre and Secondary Plant Compounds

Even though the human body cannot utilise these dietary fibres, they still play a very important role for our intestines, because our intestinal bacteria feed on them, which in turn is essential for our health. We will return to this topic later (see also Chap. 19, Microbiota and Microbiome). In addition, dietary fibres ensure that the intestines are kept "on the go", i.e. in motion. They bind water, increase stool volume and thus contribute to regular digestion.

But plant foods have even more to offer. In addition to dietary fibre, they also contain the so-called secondary plant substances. Secondary plant

© The Author(s), under exclusive license to Springer-Verlag GmbH, DE, part of Springer Nature 2023
A. Friedrich, *The Multiple Sclerosis Companion*,
https://doi.org/10.1007/978-3-662-67540-3_17

substances include, for example, the so-called polyphenols, carotenoids and flavonoids and have antioxidant and anti-inflammatory effects that also benefit us and our health. They give fruits and vegetables their colour and aroma and serve as protection for the plants, namely as a defence against pests and diseases.

17.2   Effects of the Plant-Based Diet

What effect a plant-based diet can have on the human body is what we want to look at in the following paragraphs, based on a selection of studies. We will start with two small nutritional studies, which are initially not about MS at all, but about important risk factors for vascular diseases, such as increased cholesterol and diabetes—two diseases that are known to be very widespread in all industrialised nations and cause great damage to health through heart attacks and strokes.

In the first small Canadian study with 46 participants, the effectiveness of a vegetarian, i.e. plant-based, diet was compared with the conventional cholesterol-lowering therapy (so-called statins) in adults with high blood cholesterol levels over a period of 1 month. The results showed that the cholesterol reduction was equally good in both groups, and that the plant-based diet was just as effective as the statin drug therapy.

The second small study with 74 participants dealt with diabetics and compared a diabetic group (type 2, i.e. the "acquired type" of diabetes) that received a conventional diabetes diet according to orthodox medicine for 24 weeks with a second group that received a vegetarian diet with the same number of patients. Here, the vegetarian diet was found to be even superior to the standard diabetes diet.

In these two small studies, it could thus be shown that for the two classic vascular risk factors diabetes and increased cholesterol, vegetarian nutrition was equivalent or even superior to the respective orthodox medical concept.

17.3   The "China Study"

After these studies with a small number of cases, now comes a very large, if not the largest, nutrition study on this topic: The China Study. The China Study is a huge, epidemiological study. The nutrition researcher and biochemist Prof. Dr. T. Colin Campbell, Professor of Biochemistry at Cornell University, Ithaca, NY, led this study in the 1970s and 1980s and summarised the results in his book of the same name. Such a huge study became possible after the Prime Minister of China fell ill with cancer. He then wanted a nationwide study to learn more about the causes of cancer, and so this huge study was initiated. Over a period of 27 years, a total of more than 6500 people were examined in 65 counties in China. The investigations were extensive: from blood and urine samples to food analyses and standardised interviews. In this way, enormous amounts of data were collected and more than 8000 statistically significant correlations between lifestyle, diet and diseases were recorded. What was striking, according to the author, was a strong correlation between the consumption of animal proteins and the incidence of cancer, but also of diabetes, cardiovascular diseases, obesity, autoimmune diseases and degenerative brain diseases. In contrast, a plant-based, high-fibre diet was associated with a very low incidence of these diseases. The criticism of this massive population study is that it is only correlational (i.e. determined by a probability) and not causal (determined by a cause-effect relationship). This correlation-causality dilemma is a fundamental problem of many nutrition studies. As they say in scientific jargon, "correlation does not prove causality". In nutrition studies, how do you prove that a single isolated factor really causes a single outcome? This is where animal studies come in handy, which we will come back to later. However, as you can see in the following, patterns of relationships between nutrition, lifestyle and certain diseases can be identified again and again.

17.4 China's Shift to the "Western Diet" and Its Consequences

We stay in China for the time being. China has always been known for its traditional diet. Just as the Greek physician Hippocrates did around 400 years before Christ, traditional Chinese medicine (TCM) also relies on nutrition as an important pillar of treatment. The basics of the Chinese food pyramid consist mainly of cereals, rice and additionally plenty of steamed vegetables, mushrooms, high-quality oils, little meat and fish and only very reduced milk. Sweets, bread or pastries were not common. A very interesting Chinese study from 2016 now shows that in China the change in diet away from the traditional and towards the Western diet has led to a significant increase in all Western civilisation diseases such as cardiovascular diseases, high blood pressure, lipometabolic disorders, carcinomas, diabetes and obesity.

17.5   What Can a Plant-Based Mediterranean Diet Do?

Away from the Chinese diet and towards the Mediterranean diet, which is perhaps more familiar to most of us: The following is a large meta-analysis, i.e. a statistical review of data from previous research results. In this meta-analysis, the influence of a Mediterranean diet on mortality from various diseases was investigated. For this purpose, data from 12 studies from the years 1966 to 2008 were statistically analysed in the paper published in 2008. The results showed that a Mediterranean diet led to a measurably better state of health, recognisable by a 9% reduction in cardiovascular disease mortality, a 6% reduction in cancer mortality and a 13% reduction in new cases of Parkinson's and Alzheimer's.

A recent, large US study from 2016 with 131,342 participants also showed similar results. Here, the influence of proteins was examined and the mortality under a diet with plant versus animal proteins was compared over the years 1980–2012. The results showed that animal protein consumption was associated with high cardiovascular mortality. In contrast, high consumption of plant proteins had the opposite effect and was associated with low overall mortality and particularly low cardiovascular mortality.

According to this research, it obviously makes a difference to our bodies whether we eat animal or plant proteins.

Another large Spanish study on the Mediterranean diet was conducted in 2013 with 7447 participants. All participants had an increased risk of cardiovascular disease. The question was whether the cardiovascular risk could be reduced by a high-fat or rather low-fat diet. The study design was interesting: there was a low-fat control group and a "Mediterranean group" consisting of two subgroups, both of which received a high-fat diet. To ensure that the two subgroups in the Mediterranean group also consumed fat, the participants in the first Mediterranean subgroup each received 1 litre of olive oil per week free of charge, while those in the second Mediterranean subgroup were instead provided with nuts free of charge (30 g nut mixture of walnuts, hazelnuts and almonds). The participants in the low-fat control group were not given any supplementary food. The results were impressive and spectacular for the participants in the two Mediterranean groups who ate a high-fat diet. The high-fat Mediterranean diet drastically reduced the risk of heart attack or stroke compared to the low-fat control group.

Even existing vascular damage can be reduced by a change in diet—Dr. Caldwell Esselstyn was able to show this in a small study in 1995. In patients with severe coronary artery disease, he was able to demonstrate a reduction in arteriosclerosis (i.e. a reduction in the already existing vascular calcification) and in the angiography of the coronary vessels after a change in diet with additional intake of cholesterol-lowering drugs. Similar results were obtained in a study published in the Lancet in 1990. Here, changes in lifestyle with a vegetarian diet, nicotine withdrawal, stress management training as well as light physical activity led to an improvement in the findings even in severe coronary artery disease after 1 year, even without additional intake of cholesterol-lowering drugs.

A recent Danish cohort study (i.e. an observational study that aims to uncover the relationship between certain circumstances and the occurrence of a disease) from 2017 showed that a plant-based diet with vegetables, fruits, fibre and some fish demonstrated this positive vascular effect also in strokes. So, it seems:

> The more plant-based and Mediterranean, the better—not only for the cardio-vascular system, but also for the brain!

As already mentioned, MS is on the rise, just like the typical civilisation diseases of the Western world, and there is much evidence that diet has a clear influence on civilisation diseases. Does this also apply to MS? If we know from studies on twins that only about **30%** of the risk of disease is determined **genetically,** while **70% is** determined by **environmental factors,** could lifestyle adaptation with dietary changes also be effective in MS?

Much of the research on nutrition, immune system and MS comes mainly from animal models, primarily mouse studies. When it comes to the question of how nutrition might work, interesting tracks lead to the intestine and its inhabitants, the microbiota and the microbiome. We will deal with this very new and exciting topic in the next chapter "The Intestine and Its Inhabitants".

18

The Intestine and Its Inhabitants

The role of the intestine came increasingly into the focus of medical attention at the end of the twentieth century, because it was suspected that the microorganisms of the digestive tract could have an influence on a wide variety of diseases. In the meantime, there have been numerous scientific studies on this.

But before we turn to the intestinal contents with the bacteria and the exciting findings on "microbiome research", we should first briefly look at the structure of the gastrointestinal tract.

18.1 What Does the Gastrointestinal Tract Look Like?

Let us first look at the gastrointestinal tract in the following figure for an overview (Fig. 18.1). It shows the oesophagus, which connects the mouth to the stomach, followed by the small intestine and the frame-like large intestine, which merges into the rectum and then continues to the intestinal outlet, the anus.

The human intestine is a huge organ. Consisting of both small and large intestine, it has a total length of between 5.50 and 7.50 metres and a surface area of about 32–35 square metres in adults. This corresponds to the size of quite a large room. It is really amazing that there is space for so much intestine in our stomach.

A. Friedrich, *The Multiple Sclerosis Companion*, https://doi.org/10.1007/978-3-662-67540-3_18

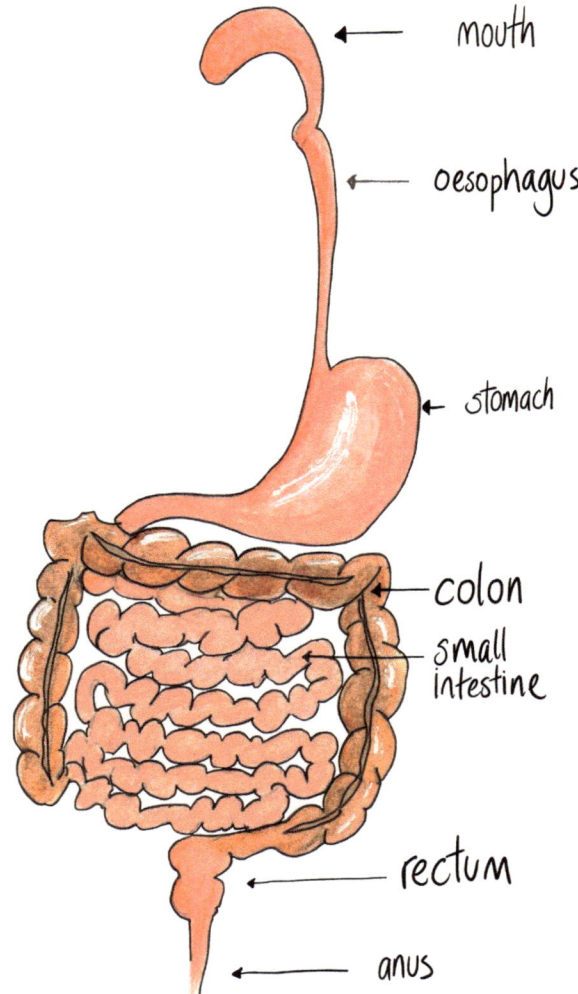

Fig. 18.1 From the mouth to the anus—a long and exciting journey

18.2   Three Layers: Mucosa, Connective Tissue and Musculature

In the cross section are three layers of the intestine: the mucosal layer, the connective tissue layer and the two-layered muscle layer (Fig. 18.2).

If we start from the inside, the so-called lumen, we first recognise the mucous membrane layer, also called mucosa. It has finger-shaped elevations, the intestinal villi, which serve to enlarge the surface. The connective tissue

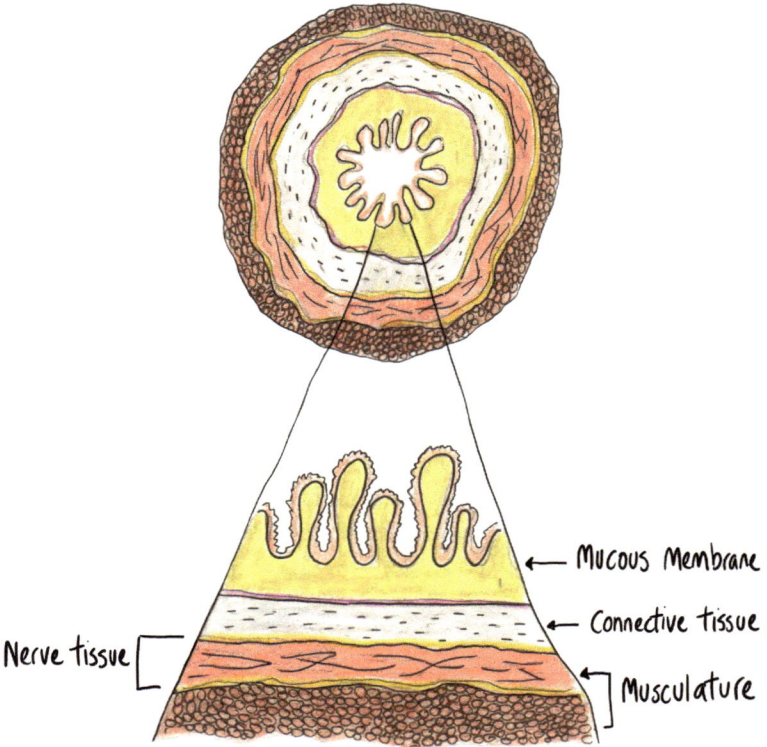

Fig. 18.2 Mucosal, connective tissue and muscle layer in cross section (top) and magnified (bottom)

layer, also called the submucosa, follows as the middle layer, and then the two-part muscle layer, muscularis, which ensures good intestinal motility.

18.3   The Intestine Has Its Own Nervous System: The "Enteric Nervous System"

Both in the connective tissue layer and in the muscle layer, there is nerve tissue as a kind of nerve plexus, the "plexus submucosus" in the connective tissue layer and the "plexus myentericus" in the muscle layer (Fig. 18.2). The nervous system of the intestine is called the "enteric nervous system". It contains more nerve cells than the spinal cord and is more like the central than the peripheral nervous system. The enteric nervous system controls intestinal movements and secretion of enzymes. But it probably has many more "communicative tasks" between the intestine and the brain that we do not yet fully see today.

18.4 The Intestine and Its Own Immune System: The "GALT"

If we look at the mucosa, i.e. the inner mucosal layer of the intestine, under microscopic magnification, we notice how much is going on there. And interestingly, we find the same players there that we already got to know at the blood–brain barrier in Chap. 3, "A Trip into Our Immune System". There are macrophages and dendritic cells as antigen-presenting cells (APCs), which are in close contact with T and B lymphocytes. Lymphoid tissues in the form of lymph follicles and lymph nodes are also present in the intestinal wall. The intestinal wall thus harbours its own local immune system, the so-called gut-associated lymphoid tissue, or "GALT" for short (Fig. 18.3).

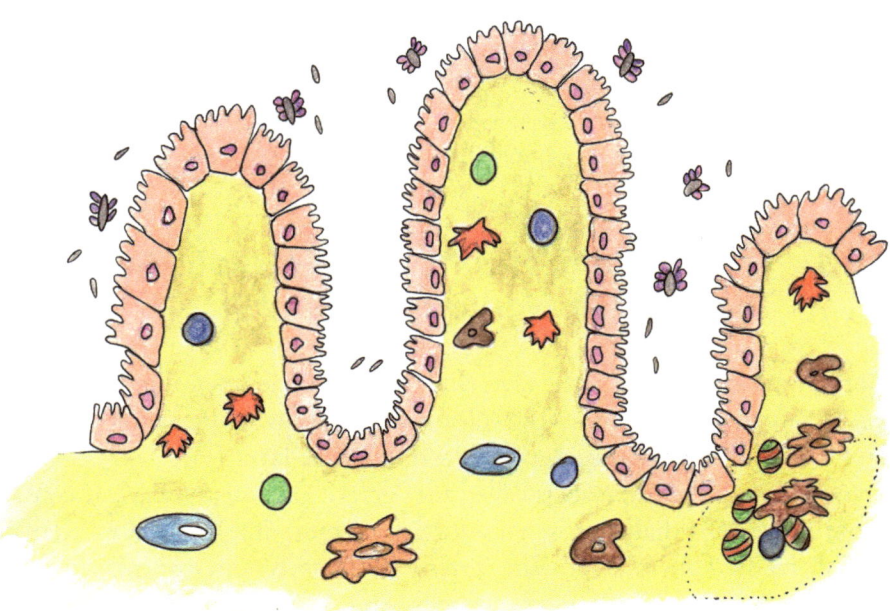

Fig. 18.3 The intestinal mucosa enlarged with "GALT"

18.5   The Intestine Has Immense Possibilities for Interaction

Just as blood and cerebrospinal fluid are only separated from each other by a thin epithelial layer at the blood–brain barrier (Chap. 5), the intestinal epithelial cells face the intestinal contents as a thin single-row cell layer towards the intestinal lumen. These contain foreign substances, food residues and bacteria. With this spatial proximity, an intensive exchange between the food residues, the bacteria and the immune system would be conceivable. And one can imagine how important the barrier function of the intestinal epithelial cells must be.

The intestine is in active exchange: it is in contact with food and the foreign substances it contains. It is in contact with the intestinal bacteria and their metabolic products. It is in contact with the immune system located in the intestinal wall, with the enteric nervous system and with the blood and lymphatic system, through which it is connected to the entire body. The intestine is therefore interconnected in many ways, which already suggests its great influence.

Now that we have learned about the structure of the gastrointestinal tract in this chapter, we will turn to the inhabitants of the intestine.

19

Microbiota and Microbiome

Now let us have a closer look at the living content of our intestines: the bacteria. Bacteria live not only in the intestine but also on the skin and the mucous membranes of the oral cavity, nasal cavity, throat and genitals. In fact, our whole body is covered with bacteria. However, the largest population of bacteria is found in the digestive tract, especially in the lower small intestine and the colon. The mass of bacteria in the intestine is about 2 kg. The sum of all bacteria in the intestine is called the intestinal microbiota. Microbiome and microbiota are two terms that are often used synonymously, but actually this is not correct. While gut microbiota refers to the totality of all microorganisms that colonise the gut, microbiome refers to the totality of all **genes** of these microorganisms. This is because the microorganisms also carry genetic information.

19.1 Bacteria in the Majority

It is an incredible thought that most cells in the human body are not human cells at all, but bacterial! These microbial cells far outnumber human cells at an estimated ratio of 10:1.

This means that there are ten times more bacterial cells than human cells in the human body!

© The Author(s), under exclusive license to Springer-Verlag GmbH, DE, part of Springer Nature 2023
A. Friedrich, *The Multiple Sclerosis Companion*,
https://doi.org/10.1007/978-3-662-67540-3_19

In numbers: There are approximately 100 billion microbial cells compared to approximately 10 billion human cells. Not only human cells contain hereditary information in the form of genes, but also bacterial cells do too. And again, there are about 150 times more bacterial genes than human genetic information in our human bodies. In addition to the bacterial cells with their genetic information, there are also some viruses and fungi that also play a role. So, it would not be surprising if this superset of cells and genes foreign to the body did not also have something to say about it. The question of who governs whom does not seem unfounded in view of such immense numbers.

19.2   Our Intestine: A Giant "Bioreactor"

We are inclined to think of bacteria as our enemies, and often the term antibiotic is mentioned in the same breath. However, we forget that humans and many bacteria actually live together symbiotically, i.e. support each other and even need each other. Imagine the human intestine as a kind of giant "bioreactor" of bacteria that supplies our body with energy. The intestinal microbiota, with its diverse genetic but also metabolic properties, helps us to generate vital nutrients from the food we eat that the human intestine could not acquire on its own. For example, some intestinal bacteria process food contents that are indigestible for humans into important vitamins and messenger substances. These include biotin, which is important for skin, hair, blood cells and nerve tissue. Also, vitamin K, which is important for blood clotting; vitamin B12 and folic acid, which are needed for DNA synthesis and repair; or messenger substances such as serotonin, which in turn influences our mood, all belong to this group. Not only vitamins and messenger substances but also short-chain fatty acids are formed from dietary fibre by the action of bacteria. The short-chain fatty acids in turn serve as an energy source for the intestinal cells and are thus important for their function such as maintaining the barrier function of the intestinal epithelial cells. The short-chain fatty acids also play a crucial role for the immune system. We will come back to this point in more detail later, when we deal specifically with studies on the intestine, the immune system and MS (Chap. 23). As you can see, the intestinal bacteria are of decisive importance for us in many respects. They influence us with their genetic information, modify our metabolism, form a barrier against pathogens, fight inflammation, detoxify foreign substances, maintain the balance in the intestine, influence our immune system and can probably do even much much more.

The gut microbiota with its diverse tasks thus represents a hidden, influential organ in the gut that stands on its own. However, this organ is not static, because it develops with us. It is subject to age-related change and can be altered by environmental influences. In the meantime, it is even assumed that every person has their own individual and unique bacterial microbiota.

But first let us look at how the microbiota develops with the microbiome in the gut.

20

How the Microbiome Develops

The life of the unborn child in the womb is still germ-free. The newborn's first contact with bacteria is during the birth process, because then it comes into contact with the mother's germs. The vaginal mucosa contains many lactobacilli, which the newborn needs to digest the mother's milk. The newborn also comes into contact with the mother's intestinal bacteria during the birth process. The next contact with bacteria is the skin of the mother's breast, which is also colonised. The child's intestine therefore first develops through contact with the mother's bacteria, which is the first "bacterial stamp" that is put on the intestine. In the course of time, other bacteria are added through nutrition and environmental contact (children like to put many things in their mouths) and gradually colonise the child's intestine. In this way, the child's increasingly complex intestinal microbiota develops. In the 2nd–4th years of life, the child's intestinal microbiota is largely similar to that of the adult intestinal colonisation. The extent to which the natural birth process and breastfeeding have an influence on the composition of the child's intestinal mucosa and the child's later immunity has not yet been conclusively clarified.

20.1 A Healthy Intestine = Eubiosis, a Diseased Intestine = Dysbiosis

The tasks of the microbiota are manifold. The bacteria are responsible for breaking down and utilising food components; they form vital vitamins and messenger substances and short-chain fatty acids such as acetate (acetic acid),

© The Author(s), under exclusive license to Springer-Verlag GmbH, DE, part of Springer Nature 2023
A. Friedrich, *The Multiple Sclerosis Companion*,
https://doi.org/10.1007/978-3-662-67540-3_20

butyrate (butyric acid) and propionate (propionic acid) from indigestible food components. They create a barrier against pathogens, fight inflammation, detoxify foreign substances and play an important role in the intestinal immune system. These intestinal bacteria are therefore real workhorses. The presence of a stable, balanced, species-rich gut microbiota that can handle these tasks is called **eubiosis**. The opposite of eubiosis is **dysbiosis**. Whereas in eubiosis germs that are useful to humans (so-called "symbionts"), germs without pathogenic significance ("commensals") and germs with pathogenic potential ("pathobionts") are in balance with each other, this balance is disturbed in dysbiosis. In dysbiosis, there is a "microbial imbalance", i.e. a pathological imbalance in the intestine with incorrect colonisation and predominance of pathobionts and restrictions in bacterial species diversity.

What causes can lead from eubiosis to dysbiosis? Ultimately, many different factors contribute. It can be the person's genetic make-up, but it can also be environmental factors and lifestyle above all.

> The influence of lifestyle becomes clear when you consider that identical twins, i.e. siblings with exactly the same genetic make-up, do not have the same microbiota. This is because our lifestyle changes the composition of our intestinal colonisation.

Antibiotic therapies, for example, destroy 90% of the bacteria in the entire body in one go, even "the good ones". And if animals such as pigs or chickens are treated with antibiotics so that they do not fall ill so easily in the cramped conditions in which they are kept, these antibiotics also end up in our food.

There is much evidence that the "Western diet" contributes to the alteration of the microbiota with restriction of bacterial biodiversity. But other factors such as stress, hygiene, infections or bacterial colonisation in early life through caesarean section, breastfeeding practices, etc. are also discussed.

But how can the intestinal bacteria actually be detected? You are about to find out in the next chapter.

21

How Bacteria Can Be Identified

In the past, bacteria were identified exclusively by growing them on culture media, and this "past" was not so long ago. Until the 1980s, cultures were set up on classical culture media, in so-called Petri dishes, and the bacteria were grown there (classical culture technique). As we know today, many microorganisms cannot be cultivated outside their habitat. They therefore remain invisible to us, yet still exist. With these classical culture methods, therefore, only a small part of the actually existing bacteria was recorded, and in this way, it was possible to detect about 100 different intestinal species, including a high proportion of so-called *E. coli* bacteria. Therefore, it was assumed for a long time that the main part of the intestinal colonisation consists of strains of *E. coli*. However, this is wrong, as we know today through newer techniques.

21.1 Microbiome Analysis by "Next-Generation Sequencing" (NGS)

The modern sequencing technique "NGS" makes it possible to capture the sum of bacteria not through the cells, but through their genetics. NGS stands for next-generation sequencing and with this technique something incredible is possible, because the entire genome, i.e. the entire genetic information, can be read in a short time.

> Through NGS, individual bacterial strains can be recorded and identified via their genes.

© The Author(s), under exclusive license to Springer-Verlag GmbH, DE, part of Springer Nature 2023
A. Friedrich, *The Multiple Sclerosis Companion*,
https://doi.org/10.1007/978-3-662-67540-3_21

Thus, not 100 bacterial species, but far more than 1000 different species could be identified by this microbiome analysis.

21.2   Species Richness of the Microbiota

With the help of NGS, statements can also be made about the species richness of the examined microbiota of a person, i.e. determinations of the qualitative composition of the microbiota. This can then be compared in a second step with a "normal collective" via a database. In this way, it can be determined whether the examined microbiota of a person corresponds to a normal bacterial composition with a high species diversity or whether it deviates from it. Such comparisons have shown that the Yanomami Indians, who live completely isolated from the Western world, have the most species-rich, variable microbiota, while the Western population has the poorest. From these results, it was concluded that Western lifestyles have a significant effect on the species richness of the human microbiota. Does the Western diet lead to microbiota depletion? And what role does a large bacterial biodiversity play in our health?

If a healthy intestine is so important and the intestinal contents with their inhabitants fulfil such essential tasks, what actually happens when you transfer microbiota? We will explore this exciting question in the next chapter, which deals with stool transplantation and its possible consequences.

22

The Stool Transplant

FMT stands for "faecal microbiota transplantation" and means stool transplantation. You are probably asking yourself, what on earth is a stool transplant? And yes, you can indeed transplant stool. The first description of stool transplantation dates back to ancient China in the fourth century AD, and it was done for severe diarrhoea and food poisoning.

In modern times, there is also a reason for performing stool transplantation. It is performed in cases of therapy-resistant infection with a certain disease-causing bacterium called "*Clostridium difficile*". A *Clostridium difficile* infection, known as CDI for short, can lead to severe, life-threatening diarrhoea. The disease is caused by an overgrowth of infectious *Clostridium difficile* bacteria in the intestine, which leads to dysbiosis (Chap. 20) by displacement of the usual bacteria in the intestine. The severe intestinal infection is initially treated with antibiotics. However, if even repeated antibiotic treatments do not lead to an improvement of the life-threatening condition, stool transplantation is performed as the last therapeutic measure. In the case of *Clostridium difficile* infection, it has an extraordinarily high cure rate of 60–90%, so what sounds rather unpleasant at first can have a life-saving effect. The transplanted healthy microbiota of a donor ensures that the *Clostridium difficile* germ is relegated to its place and a balance is restored in the intestine (eubiosis).

© The Author(s), under exclusive license to Springer-Verlag GmbH, DE, part of Springer
Nature 2023
A. Friedrich, *The Multiple Sclerosis Companion*,
https://doi.org/10.1007/978-3-662-67540-3_22

22.1   FMT and Practical Implementation

How should one imagine such a transplantation in practice? In stool transplantation, frozen stool from a healthy person (obtained from a National Stool Transplant Register, for example) is thawed, dissolved in NaCl (i.e. a saline solution), filtered and then introduced into the patient's intestine with the help of a colonoscopy. Recently, as an alternative to microbiota transfer by colonoscopy, there is also the option of swallowing a capsule containing the substrate. After a successful microbiota transfer, one can then see in the control colonoscopy that the intestine has recovered and the mucosa looks shiny and healthy again. If the therapy is successful, the microbiome analysis shows a great diversity of species again due to the transplanted new bacteria.

22.2   FMT and Consequences

However, one must be warned against the reckless use of such procedures. Although this measure is very effective, there may also be unforeseeable risks associated with it, as you can see from the following case report. The report describes the case of a patient with refractory CDI infection who received a stool transplant from her 16-year-old, severely overweight daughter. The transplant was successful because after the stool transfer, the life-threatening Clostridia infection healed, but the previously slim patient suddenly became severely overweight, like her daughter.

A comparable result is shown by a study with stool transplantation in animal experiments with mice. Human intestinal bacteria were transferred to germ-free mice raised. The human stool donors were identical twins, i.e. they had the same genetic make-up. However, one twin was very overweight, while the other was of normal weight. After the stool transplantation from human to mouse, in the first case, the mouse also became overweight, and in the second case, the mouse remained thin. There was a second part of the experiment; here, the mice were put back together in a common cage immediately after the transplantation. Surprisingly, neither mouse then gained weight. Because mice eat the faeces of their conspecifics, they can obviously exchange their microbiota, and they thus apparently performed their own "reverse transplantation". Such exciting findings of stool transplantation show how much "information" is in the gut and the microbiota.

We will look at what influence the intestine and its microbiota have on the immune system and thus could possibly also have on MS using some animal experiments in the following chapter.

23

The Bowel and MS: What Does Scientific Research Say?

In the following pages, we will look at a selection of studies on the intestine and MS, or rather nutrition, microbiome, immune system and MS, because we want to go back to our initial question: Does a lifestyle adjustment with dietary changes have a positive effect not only on diabetes, cholesterol, metabolism disorders or cardiovascular diseases, but also on MS?

On the subject of "bowel and MS", there is a study by Levinthal and colleagues from 2013, who first of all found that of 218 MS patients examined, two-thirds complained of various gastrointestinal complaints. Obviously, this is a widespread problem. Since I have been aware of this study, I specifically ask about it during the MS consultation and can confirm that many MS patients do indeed report complaints in this area when asked.

In contrast to this study, most of the studies presented below are animal studies that specifically shed light on the gut, the immune system and MS. In the process, you will learn some names of bacteria that are hard to pronounce, let alone remember. These include candidates such as *Bacteroides fragilis*, various lactobacilli, *Prevotella histicola*, Butyricimonas, Methanobrevibacter and many more. There are well over 1000 species of bacteria in the gut. They are classified into different bacterial strains, with each strain being further subdivided into many different families and genera. The most common bacterial strains found in the colon, with over 90%, are the Bacteroidetes and the Firmicutes.

© The Author(s), under exclusive license to Springer-Verlag GmbH, DE, part of Springer Nature 2023
A. Friedrich, *The Multiple Sclerosis Companion*,
https://doi.org/10.1007/978-3-662-67540-3_23

23.1   Animal MS Studies on Mice: "EAE"

Before we start with the various animal studies, one more important piece of information. As in many areas of preclinical research, mice are primarily used for animal experiments in MS and microbiome research. The experimental model used for MS is a mouse model with the so-called EAE. The abbreviation stands for "experimental autoimmune encephalomyelitis". This is an experimentally induced MS-like disease in mice. EAE is a T lymphocyte-mediated autoimmune disease of the mouse, and, as in MS, demyelinating lesions occur in the central nervous system. These demyelinating lesions then lead to neurological deficits typical of MS. In the following, let us look at the results of the studies like individual pieces of a jigsaw puzzle which, in the end, provide an overall picture.

23.2   Does MS Start in the Gut?

In 2017, a research group found that the intestines of mice with MS showed pathological changes even before the central nervous system was affected.

> Histologically (i.e. in the microscopic examination), these changes were already detectable in the intestine even before the MS-typical demyelination was recognisable in the brain—an indication that intestinal health plays a central role.

Even before the clinical symptoms of the experimentally induced MS disease in mice occurred, an immune reaction with antibody formation against the nerve tissue in the intestine of the animals could already be detected. In the intestinal wall, there was a loss of nerve cells with scarring, and, correspondingly, weakened intestinal musculature with reduced intestinal motility was observed in these mice. Surprisingly, the antibodies against the nerve tissue could be detected not only in the intestine, but also in the blood of the MS-affected mice. Does MS start in the gut?

23.3   Gut Bacteria and MS

A study conducted by the Max Planck Institute for Neurobiology in Munich in 2011 showed that the intestine plays a significant role in the development of MS. Using genetically modified mice raised completely germ-free (so-called "germ-free" mice), it was shown that the mice did not develop an autoimmune disease when the intestine was sterile, i.e. germ-free. From this observation, it was concluded that bacterial intestinal colonisation is a prerequisite for the development of demyelination in the central nervous system. A study from 2009 on the experimental MS model of the mouse had already shown that antibiotic-pre-treated mice with a significantly reduced intestinal microbiota showed a weakened or delayed course of the MS disease. Both studies point to the importance of the gut in disease development.

An interesting study on twins from 2017 showed similar results. 34 identical and thus genetically identical twin pairs were compared in this study. One twin was healthy, and the other had MS. The pairs of twins were first compared with regard to their microbiota. Subsequently, a stool transplantation (FMT) was performed from each of the twins to germ-free mice. The mice that had received the microbiota of the diseased twins developed MS significantly more often than those that had received the microbiota of the healthy twins. The colleagues also concluded from this observation that the human intestinal contents must contain components that promote the onset of the disease.

What is the potential of the gut? To what extent does the microbiota of MS sufferers differ from that of healthy people, and is there a specific intestinal germ that can be held responsible for MS? Many studies have dealt with this question. In the study on twins described above, in which the microbiota of identical twin pairs was compared before stool transplantation, no differences were found between the microbiota of healthy people and those with MS. In contrast, a study from Harvard in 2016 came to a different conclusion. In this study, the microbiota of 60 MS patients and 43 healthy volunteers was examined and the bacterial composition was compared in both the healthy volunteers and MS patients. The microbiota of MS patients contained more bacteria called Methanobrevibacter and Akkermansia, but less Butyricimonas. The microbiota of healthy people contained the opposite, little Methanobrevibacter and Akkermansia and especially a lot of Butyricimonas. It is interesting that the two types of bacteria, which were found particularly frequently in the intestines of MS patients, are said to have pro-inflammatory properties. Methanobrevibacter, for example, is known to have pro-inflammatory effects through its ability to activate pro-inflammatory cells and dendritic antigen-presenting cells (APCs). Akkermansia also correlates with pro-inflammatory effects through upregulation of antigen-presenting receptors on B and T lymphocytes. Butyricimonas, on the other hand, which was found in increased numbers in the microbiota of healthy individuals, is attributed with anti-inflammatory influences. This is because Butyricimonas produces the short-chain fatty acid butyrate, which serves as an energy source for the intestinal epithelial cells and is thus important for a healthy intestinal mucosa and the maintenance of the intestinal barrier function. However, short-chain fatty acids also have a direct dampening effect on the immune system, as we will see later. There are also many other papers that have looked at the differences in the microbiota between healthy people and people with MS.

> However, no "concrete MS germ" has been found so far. Nevertheless, the intestinal colonisation seems to have an important influence on the function of the immune system and the development of MS.

That the microbiota obviously intervenes decisively in our immune system and that there is an intensive interplay between the intestinal bacteria and the immune system became clear not only from the inflammation-firing influences of Akkermansia and Methanobrevibacter described above. Pro-inflammatory influences on the immune system have also been identified in other bacteria. For example, a study by Ivanov and colleagues in 2009 showed that overgrowth of the intestine in mice with so-called segmented filamentous bacteria (SFB) led to the increased production of inflammation-firing Th17 cells in the intestinal wall, which was then in turn accompanied by inflammation. Some specific bacterial species that can activate autoimmune CNS diseases (such as SFB, Akkermansia or Methanobrevibacter) and others that ameliorate the disease (such as Butyricimonas, *Bacteroides fragilis*, Prevotella or some lactobacilli) have now been identified. However, it is now also known that not only the bacteria influence the immune cells, but also the immune cells influence the composition of the microbiota. You see how complex this interaction in the gut seems to be and it is still not completely understood.

23.4 The Metabolic Products of the Bacteria and MS

While the initial focus of the studies was on the intestine and its bacterial composition, in recent years, there has been increasing evidence that not only the bacteria themselves, but also their metabolic products can have a decisive influence on the immune system. What do bacteria produce, for example, from the food we give them? The realisation that we should not only look at bacteria and their biodiversity, but also at their metabolic products, has led to the exciting field of so-called metabolomics.

23.5 High-Fibre Diet: Energy Source for the Intestinal Cells

As early as 2004, a paper described that high-fibre diets produce short-chain fatty acids through the action of bacteria in the intestine. Acetate (acetic acid) is the most produced short-chain fatty acid (60%), followed by propionate (propionic acid) with 25% and butyrate (butyric acid) with 15%. It is described that more than 95% of the short-chain fatty acids produced by the bacteria are needed in the colon itself. They are absorbed by the intestinal epithelial cells and used by them as an energy source. Here, butyrate in particular is considered the preferred energy source. The short-chain fatty acids from a high-fibre diet thus have an important influence on the intestinal cells and their function. A new study from 2019 on MS patients has now been able to show that precisely these important short-chain fatty acids are diminished in patients with multiple sclerosis.

23.6 Short-Chain Fatty Acids and Immune System

An exciting paper on the topic of fatty acids and their influence on the immune system was published in 2015 by Professor Haghikia's research group from Bochum, Germany. They investigated the influence of different fatty acids on the immune system in cultures and in the mouse model. Cultures with naive T lymphocytes were set up in the laboratory. As you have already heard (Chap. 3), naive T lymphocytes are not yet differentiated T lymphocytes that can transform into pro-inflammatory (Th1, Th17) or anti-inflammatory (T-reg) T lymphocytes depending on the stimulus. In the experiment, different fatty acids were added to these naive T lymphocytes and the reaction of the T lymphocytes was examined. If the short-chain fatty acid propionate (propionic acid) was added, the naive T lymphocytes converted more into the anti-inflammatory T-regulatory lymphocytes (T-reg). However, when they added the long-chain fatty acid laurate (lauric acid), the naive T cells converted into the pro-inflammatory Th1 and Th17 lymphocytes. This experiment was then repeated in the animal model on mice, and the same thing was seen. If the mice were fed a diet containing propionate, increased T-reg could be detected in the intestinal mucosa. In addition, the mice showed a milder disease course with reduced demyelination and less axonal nerve damage. In contrast, when the mice were fed a laurate-containing diet, the animals showed the opposite, namely increased inflammation-firing Th1 and Th17 cells in the gut and increased disease activity in the central nervous system. In complementary metabolic studies in 2018, another detrimental effect of laurate-rich diets was found: When mice were fed the fatty acid laurate, there was a regular decrease in the important short-chain fatty acids acetate, butyrate and propionate in the intestine.

> So, at least in the animal model, there seems to be a direct connection between the type of fatty acids ingested and the immune response in the intestine or brain, with a corresponding influence on the course of the disease.

23.7   Nutrition and Microbiota

Now you have received important new information about fatty acids and their influence on the immune system and are probably wondering which fatty acids are actually found in which products. It is interesting that the medium- and long-chain fatty acids, e.g. palmitate and laurate, are concentrated in products of the so-called Western diet, while the short-chain fatty acids which nourish and protect the intestinal epithelium are mainly found in high-fibre, plant-based foods.

So, let us look at some more studies that deal with the direct influence of diet on the gut and its microbiota in mice and humans.

In a paper from 2009, it was described that a change from a plant-based, fibre-rich diet to a high-fat and high-sugar diet, such as the "Western diet", led to a change in the microbiota and its metabolic products in mice within 1 day. This finding was also confirmed in humans. A study from 2014 also showed in the human intestine that the microbiota adapts very quickly to a change in diet. The composition of the microbiota differed depending on the diet, and it was also recognisable whether the person consumed more meat or more plant-based food. The microbiota can obviously adapt quickly to the food it receives or in other words:

> Food shapes the microbiota.

An Australian review from 2016 vividly summarises how diet influences gut bacteria and their metabolites and modulates the immune system. Here, too, it can be read that plant-based, whole-food, high-fibre diets influence the intestinal microbiota and its species diversity (eubiosis). Bacteria (especially

Bacteroidetes) produce short-chain fatty acids such as acetate, butyrate and propionate via fermentation of fibre-rich indigestible food residues. Short-chain fatty acids, as you now know, in turn have an anti-inflammatory effect, as they stimulate the proliferation of T-reg lymphocytes. Short-chain fatty acids, especially butyrate, are also a source of energy for the intestinal epithelial cells and thus important for the barrier function of the intestinal mucosa. As already described, a deficiency of short-chain fatty acids in the intestine has been found in MS patients, and indeed work from 2017 and 2018 was also able to demonstrate an increased permeability of the intestinal wall in MS patients with relapsing-remitting MS (RRMS).

23.8 Back to the Western Diet

As we have now seen from many studies, the gut microbiota is not something static, but evolves with us and can be changed by environmental influences. But it is not only our choice of fats that can modulate the microbiota and our immune system. In the animal model, the same was shown for increased salt and sugar consumption, because here, too, inflammatory influences (via activation of Th17 cells with the release of pro-inflammatory messenger substances) could be objectified. With high salt consumption, changes in the microbiota with reduction of the important lactobacilli were determined and a negative influence on the course of the disease in MS patients was described. However, in addition to the inflammation-firing environmental factors, protective factors that calm the immune system were also found (Chap. 24).

23.9 Many Studies, Many Pieces of the Puzzle

At the moment, these are just pieces of the puzzle and there are still many missing pieces until the finished picture. Diseases for which a connection to the intestinal microbiota is now seen are increasing more and more because the dysbiosis of the gut seems to be associated with many other chronic diseases. Even though we are still far from understanding all the connections, there is growing evidence that environmental factors and especially our dietary choices change the microbiota, which in turn has an influence on the immune system that goes far beyond the gut.

23.10   Just Give It a Try

And here we come full circle to the observations from my everyday practice:

> Nutrition works!

It seems that a plant-based, whole-food, high-fibre diet triggers anti-inflammatory effects with the help of the intestinal bacteria, nourishes the intestinal epithelial cells and thus ensures a good barrier function of the intestinal epithelium. In contrast, the widespread "Western diet" with many long-chain fatty acids and trans-fats, and high sugar and salt content, seems to trigger inflammation-firing processes via the microbiota and its metabolic products, with subsequent effects that go far beyond the intestine.

So, what is wrong with trying a plant-based, high-fibre diet? How about just giving it a try? There are countless, extremely tasty, plant-based recipes and you will find some in Chap. 25. Especially those who suffer from the chronic fatigue syndrome (fatigue syndrome) know very well the high degree of suffering associated with it. Since there is no conventional medical therapy available so far, those affected should try this dietary optimisation, proceed in stages, give themselves some time and observe the progress.

23.11   Propionate: As a Food Supplement

The short-chain fatty acid propionate is also available for purchase as a food supplement. Since a deficiency of short-chain fatty acids in the intestine has been found in MS patients, propionate has been recommended for some time now in a daily dose of two capsules (500 mg) by colleagues in Bochum, Germany.

Propionate may be useful as an add-on therapy, and further studies on its effect in relapsing-remitting MS (RRMS) are eagerly awaited.

However, in my opinion, it is a supplement and not an alternative to a healthy, plant-based diet, which is more than an isolated fatty acid. Plant-based, whole food contains more. On the one hand, it contains dietary fibre, from which our intestinal bacteria produce various short-chain fatty acids (acetate, butyrate and propionate), which in turn nourish the intestinal epithelium and modulate the immune system. On the other hand, vegetables and fruits contain phytochemicals that help plants defend themselves against disease, and they have antioxidant and anti-inflammatory effects. All of these together make up the healthfulness of the plant-based diet and thus cannot be replaced by a single isolated short-chain fatty acid in tablet form.

Further therapeutic possibilities in the future could also lie in the use of probiotics. Probiotics are living bacteria that can support the resident intestinal bacteria. In a study from 2018, immunomodulatory effects on antigen-presenting cells (APCs) were demonstrated in MS patients taking a probiotic containing lactobacilli. Further studies on the influence of probiotics are also eagerly awaited.

Before we get to the "action plan", which contains suggestions on how you can now put what you have read into practice, we will take a small diversion via vitamin D, which has already been mentioned several times.

24

Vitamin D: Sense and Nonsense

Sunlight and vitamin D came into focus early on as possible environmental factors influencing MS, after it was established that the frequency of multiple sclerosis increases with distance from the equator. There are many different study results on vitamin D and its effect, some of which differ from each other. Although sufficiently large, so-called double-blind, placebo-controlled studies are lacking, there are many indications that vitamin D has a positive influence on the immune system.

24.1   What Vitamin D Can Do

For a long time, when people thought of vitamin D, it was only thought of in terms of bone metabolism. But vitamin D takes on many more tasks in our body than just absorbing calcium from the intestines and incorporating it into the bones. There are studies that have shown that vitamin D lowers the risk of cardiovascular disease, reduces blood pressure and risk of diabetes, offers a protective effect against carcinomas (especially breast and colon carcinomas) and helps reduce bacterial and viral infection risks. Further studies show that vitamin D, through its influence on Th17 lymphocytes and antigen-presenting dendritic cells (Chap. 3), downregulates inflammation-firing processes in the immune system. This effect makes vitamin D interesting for autoimmune diseases, and there are indeed studies that showed that higher vitamin D levels in the serum correlated with a lower risk of MS.

© The Author(s), under exclusive license to Springer-Verlag GmbH, DE, part of Springer Nature 2023
A. Friedrich, *The Multiple Sclerosis Companion*,
https://doi.org/10.1007/978-3-662-67540-3_24

The finding that practically all body cells have vitamin D receptors already indicates that the effect of vitamin D must be more diverse than previously assumed. Vitamin D receptors have also been found on immune cells. Vitamin D influences numerous metabolic processes and activates more than 1000 genes in various tissues of our body. But before we get to the mode of action, let us first take a look at where vitamin D actually comes from.

24.2   Where Vitamin D Comes from

First of all, vitamin D is not a real vitamin at all. Vitamins are substances that the body needs but cannot produce itself, which is why vitamins have to be taken in with food. This does not apply to vitamin D, however, because our body produces about 90% of vitamin D itself. Vitamin D can also be taken in with food, but this only covers a small part (about 10% of the daily requirement). In addition, only very few foods contain vitamin D; these are mainly fatty foods such as herring, mackerel, salmon, tuna, liver, egg yolk and certain mushrooms.

> By far, the largest part of vitamin D in our body is produced by the skin, and therefore vitamin D is not actually a vitamin.

It is the precursor of a hormone, a so-called prohormone, which is converted via intermediate steps to the active hormone calcitriol. We will take a closer look at this process in the following section.

24.3   In-House Production

The production of vitamin D in our skin is triggered by sunlight, or more precisely by the effect of the sun's UV-B rays. When UV-B light hits **bare** skin, it triggers a photochemical reaction in which the 7-dehydrocholesterol present in the skin is converted into vitamin D3 (cholecalciferol). However, this vitamin D3 is initially only a precursor, a prohormone, and not yet active. It must first be "switched on" by conversion steps in the liver and kidney (Fig. 24.1).

First, it goes from the skin via the blood bound to transport proteins and then to the liver. Once it reaches the liver, it is converted into an intermediate stage, 25-hydroxy-vitamin D, also called **calcidiol.**

> Calcidiol is the storage form of vitamin D. Incidentally, it is also measured in the laboratory to determine the vitamin D reserves in the body.

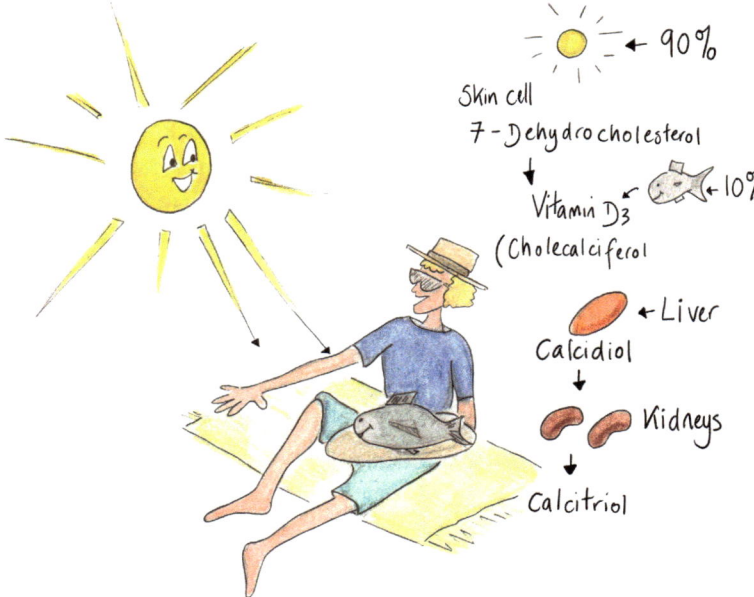

Fig. 24.1 Vitamin D production: 90% sun, 10% food

From the liver, it continues to the kidneys, where the calcidiol is converted one last time to **calcitriol** (1,25-dihydroxy-vitamin D).

Calcitriol is then ultimately the biologically active ("armed") D hormone.

The hormone exerts its actual effect via a binding site on the cells, the so-called vitamin D receptor (VDR) which is found on almost all body cells. By binding calcitriol to the receptor, numerous metabolic processes are influenced. But we will come back to the effect of the D hormone later.

Let us summarise here that the production of the hormone is a complex pathway involving several organs of the body, and sun exposure plays a very crucial role in its production.

24.4 Own Production Has a Hard Time in the Northern Climes

But watch out: Everything that gets between the skin and the sky, such as clouds, shadows, glass, sunscreen and clothing, reduces or prevents the formation of D3 hormones in the skin. Window glass, for example, absorbs practically all UV-B components in sunlight. A sunscreen with factor 8 already reduces the formation of D3 in the skin by at least 95%. Since most of us spend more time indoors than outdoors in everyday life and have already put on sunscreen when leaving the house in the sunshine, the D3 hormone production in our skin does not have it easy.

The situation is aggravated by the fact that the intensity of the UV-B rays in sunlight varies greatly from region to region. This is because the UV-B component depends on the angle of incidence of the sun's rays and the height of the sun. For sufficient vitamin D production, the angle of incidence of the sun's rays on the earth must be steeper than 35 degrees, which in the northern hemisphere is only the case between April and October. For example, in winter north of the 51st parallel, D3 can hardly be formed in the skin even at midday, whereas south of the 37th parallel (Sicily), sufficient production is possible all year round. Germany, for example, where I live, lies on the 51st parallel. This means that here, as in many other European countries and the UK, the UV-B component of the sun's radiation is extremely weak in winter. This is why there is a widespread vitamin D deficiency in our regions.

To make matters worse, as we age, the skin's 7-dehydrocholesterol content decreases and with it the ability to make vitamin D3.

> That means we need vitamin D! There are three ways to do this: large amounts of fatty fish, sun and vitamin D supplements.

24.5 Let Us Start with the Sun

The UV-B component of the sun's rays varies according to the season, time of day and cloud cover. The best time of day for sunbathing for the purpose of D3 production is midday, when the sun is at its highest. Under optimal conditions, a completely uncovered, light-skinned body can **produce** about 1000 IU of vitamin D3 **per minute** (IU stands for International Units) for about 10–15 min if the UV-B level is high enough. After these 10–15 min, the 7-dehydrocholesterol in the skin available for vitamin D3 production is used up. After that, no more vitamin D3 is produced in the exposed areas. At most, a sunburn will occur. So, on a nice sunny day, 10,000–15,000 IU of vitamin D3 could be produced by the body on its own during a 10–15-min sunbathing under optimal conditions. But in our daily lives, we would hardly ever get the chance to stand naked in the sun for 10–15 min! But this is not necessary, because every little exposure to the sun counts. Exposing the face, hands and forearms, which corresponds to about 5% of the body's surface, is enough at midday on a sunny summer day to produce about 500–750 IU of vitamin D3 after about 10–15 min of sun exposure (without sunscreen!). And again, as a reminder: If more is to be produced, more clothing must be removed, but not more time spent in the sun.

24.6 From the Sun to Vitamin D Administration (Vitamin D Substitution)

In our latitudes, the sun is not enough for most of the year because of the lack of UV-B, and the vitamin D requirement cannot be met through food, because we cannot eat that much fatty fish. So, the only option is additional substitution. And this is where the difficulty begins, because there are very different recommendations and ideas about daily requirements and target values for vitamin D. The "blood marker" for vitamin D status is the concentration of 25-hydroxy-vitamin D (calcidiol) in the blood. Calcidiol is the storage form of vitamin D in the body. Since the biologically active form of vitamin D, calcitriol (1,25-dihydroxy-vitamin D), is difficult to measure because it is present in lower concentrations in the blood and is subject to greater fluctuations, the storage form is determined in the blood. This value allows more reliable statements about the vitamin D reserves in the body.

24.7 About Calcidiol Units and Standard Values

It is confusing that there are different units for determining calcidiol in the blood. In Germany, for example, ng/mL (nanogram per millilitre) is usually used, but sometimes nmol/L (nanomole per litre) is also given. The conversion factor for this is 2.5 nmol/L = 1 ng/mL, so, e.g. 75 nmol/L = 30 ng/mL.

Opinions differ on the question of what is normal and what is deficiency. In the laboratory with which we work, normal values of 10–120 ng/mL are given for calcidiol, together with the note that "the concentration is subject to seasonal fluctuations with a minimum in winter and a maximum in autumn". The literature gives different values, mostly between 30 and 100 ng/mL (= 75–250 nmol/L) as the target value. However, if there is already disagreement about the target value, it is clear that there can be no clear statement about the daily intake dose either.

24.8   Which Vitamin D?

The question of which vitamin D should be taken is easier to answer: it should be vitamin D3, i.e. cholecalciferol, i.e. the prohormone that is also produced in the body by sunlight through self-production in the skin.

- The dosage of vitamin D3 is given in International Units (IU). Here, 25 µg corresponds to 1000 IU.
- Important: Vitamin D3 is a fat-soluble vitamin. Since it is therefore only absorbed in the presence of fats, it must be taken with a meal so that it can be absorbed in the best possible way!

There are vitamin D3 preparations in a wide variety of dosages, for example 1000 IU, 2500 IU, 5000 IU, 10,000 IU, 20,000 IU and more.

24.9   How Much Vitamin D3 for Which Target Value?

And now for the more difficult question: How much vitamin D3 should be taken in order to aim for which target value? There are very different statements on this in the literature. The German Nutrition Society (DGE), for example, assumes a target value in the blood of 20 ng/mL and recommends 800 IU (=20 µg) vitamin D3 per day if the body does not produce it itself. Internationally, a level of at least 30 ng/mL is often considered optimal and values below 10 ng/mL correspond to a severe deficiency. There are very different indications of target values, although these usually range from 30 to over 100 ng/mL. Higher target values naturally require higher daily doses, and so different experts recommend very different daily doses of vitamin D3 accordingly. You will find daily dose recommendations for healthy adults in the literature that can be as high as 4000 IU/day or even higher. If you consider that our body is able to produce 10,000–15,000 IU of vitamin D3 on its own within 10–15 min, the concern about overdose seems to be put into perspective in these dose ranges. According to a risk assessment by an American research group, doses of up to 10,000 IU per day are considered safe for healthy adults. The European Food Safety Authority (EFSA) states up to 4000 IU vitamin D3 per day without evidence of harmful effects.

But do the same recommendations also apply to existing diseases, e.g. auto-immune diseases? After what has been described so far, you can imagine that there are no uniform recommendations on this.

You will find many studies in the literature that point to the importance of vitamin D. For example, there are studies that could show that higher vitamin D levels in the serum are associated with a lower risk of MS. Such correlations have also been found in other chronic diseases, for example in various cancers or also depression. In summary, however, the question of who should take how much vitamin D cannot be answered uniformly and has not been con-clusively clarified. Ultimately, controlled studies with large numbers of cases are lacking. Factors such as the initial vitamin D level, the time of year, the frequency of "being in the sun", but also concomitant diseases play a role in the individual selection of the dose. In the case of regular higher vitamin D intake, laboratory tests should also be carried out to check the calcium level.

24.10   Effects of Vitamin D
on the Immune System

In recent years, several studies have shown that vitamin D has a significant immunomodulatory and immunoregulatory influence on different areas of our immune system. For example, it was found that a high dose of vitamin D3 of 5000–10,000 IU/day led to a significant increase in the anti-inflammatory messenger substance interleukin-10 (IL-10) and a decrease in the inflammation-firing Th17 cells.

For vitamin D to work, it must bind to a receptor, the vitamin D receptor (VDR). After binding to this receptor, vitamin D is transported into the cell nucleus. There, the vitamin D complex reacts directly with the DNA and changes the transcription of various hormone-sensitive genes with a corre-sponding biological effect. Thus, vitamin D can activate several hundred genes in the body in various organs and tissues. Vitamin D receptors are present on many cells in our body, including immune cells. An important site of action of vitamin D is the **dendritic cell (DC)**, which you know as the antigen-presenting cell (APC) in Chap. 3. Vitamin D has a strong influence on the development and maturation of various subgroups of dendritic cells and also on their function. Dendritic cells (DCs) are highly specialised antigen-presenting cells (APCs) that are very important for triggering T- and B-cell activation and thus initiating an inflammatory immune process. Vitamin D intervenes in this process. It can influence the dendritic cells, to reprogramme them and to change their behaviour in such a way that so-called tolerogenic dendritic cells are created, which lose their ability to activate Th1 and Th17 cells; instead, T-reg (T-regulatory cells) are increasingly stimulated. If we consider that in MS, the T-regulatory cells are reduced or less functional, resulting in a relative predominance of Th1 and Th17 cells, this immuno-modulatory effect of vitamin D seems significant.

24.11   Effect of the Sun

Apart from the described vitamin D effect, there is evidence that sun exposure also affects vitamin D independently in changing the immune response. A case study from the Karolinska Institute in Sweden with more than 1000 MS patients investigated the relationship between disease risk, sun exposure and vitamin D levels. They found that the disease risk was twice as high with low sun exposure and that sun exposure had its own, vitamin D-independent protective factors. Comparable findings were also confirmed in work with UV-B light in the EAE animal model of MS.

24.12   Current Vitamin D Study

There are many studies and still many unanswered questions about vitamin D and MS. The studies to date have often only been conducted with small numbers of cases, different target parameters and different doses, which is why supplementary clinical studies with larger numbers of cases are needed.

In 2012, a multicentre, randomised, double-blind vitamin D study was therefore planned. The study included MS patients who had a relapsing-remitting MS (RRMS) or a clinically isolated syndrome (CIS). All patients were on uniform immunomodulatory treatment, in this case interferon-beta 1b. The aim was to find out whether vitamin D reduces the disease activity of MS and which dose is necessary for this. One group received a high dose of vitamin D (20,400 IU) every second day and the other a low dose (400 IU every second day), and the effect was monitored by relapse rate, disability progression and MRI trajectories over 18 months. The results were published in 2020. Both vitamin D doses were well tolerated and showed no side effects. No safety risks were observed in the high-dose group either. However, there was no difference in the two therapy arms studied with regard to the investigated target parameters of relapse rate, disability progression and MRI activity. The question that arose after evaluation was whether this study with a total of 41 patients had been conducted with too low a number of cases to show possible differences.

This example clearly shows how difficult it is to implement such studies. It is important to recruit a large group of patients, if possible, under the same MS therapy, as otherwise there is no good comparability. Thus, vitamin D studies with a higher number of cases will also be necessary in the future. So much for vitamin D at this point.

And now, as already announced, to use the momentum, we come to the action plan, the practical part of this companion, where you will get suggestions on how to put what you have read into practice. Let us go!

25

Action Plan and Recipes to Follow

"Plant-based, high in fibre and good oils and a little fish, but no sugar, no meat and then as little wheat as possible …"—how is that supposed to work? Is eating still fun then?

25.1 Plant-Based Does Not Mean: No More Meat!

Do not worry, it is not about giving up meat forever, but above all about balance. The pleasure of eating should not be lost at all! And believe me, you can prepare fantastic, plant-based dishes without the feeling of "missing out" (Fig. 25.1).

Also, "plant-**based**" does not mean completely vegetarian. Instead of daily meat consumption, the goal is a shift towards more vegetables, more fibre, more whole grains and more good oils, so that meat becomes more of a side dish. You may find after a short time that even two meat portions a month are enough and fish can be added once or twice a week instead. Let us remember the "Blue Zones", the areas where there are far fewer chronic diseases. In all Blue Zones, seasonal, local vegetables with good oils form the basis of the diet.

> If you make plants the main dish and fish and especially meat the side dish, you are on the right track. Because the dose is the poison.

© The Author(s), under exclusive license to Springer-Verlag GmbH, DE, part of Springer Nature 2023
A. Friedrich, *The Multiple Sclerosis Companion*,
https://doi.org/10.1007/978-3-662-67540-3_25

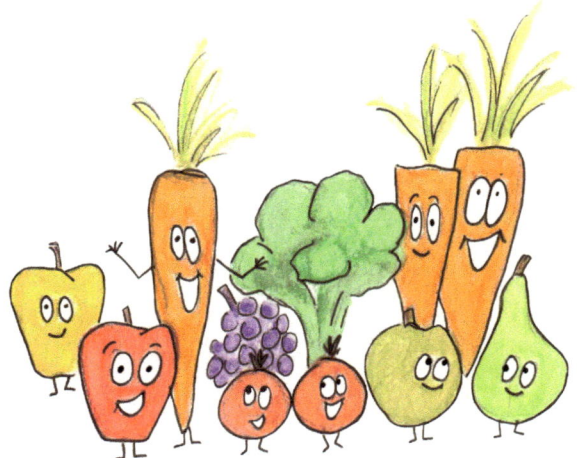

Fig. 25.1 Vegetarian diversity

And if meat, then preferably good meat from free-range organic grazing animals, which have therefore also eaten well and plant-based.

25.2   Our Attitude Is Crucial

The attitude with which we approach dietary change and the language we use are essential for success. Letting go of old habits and adopting new ones require motivation:

> Motivation to stay healthy, motivation to become healthy or motivation to stabilise the state of health.

25.3   High-Fibre Plant-Based with Good Oils Is Key!

In the following, I will give you an overview of recommended foods. You will also get a list of products that should be avoided or at least reduced if possible. This list is only a selection to get a feel for a high-fibre, plant-based diet. It does not claim to be complete.

25.4   What You Should Eat

Vegetables (rich in fibre and colourful due to secondary plant compounds)

For example, broccoli, spinach, Brussels sprouts, kale, cauliflower, white cabbage, pointed cabbage, red cabbage, sauerkraut, fennel, courgettes, leeks, onions, avocado, olives, carrots, tomatoes, beetroot, peppers, radishes, aubergines, pumpkin, cucumbers and asparagus

Legumes (high in fibre and protein)

For example, beans, peas, lentils and chickpeas (hummus)

Salad (low in calories, high in fibre and full of vitamins and minerals)

All kinds of lettuce

Mushrooms (source of protein and ideal alternative to meat)

For example, oyster mushrooms, mushrooms, shiitake, porcini mushrooms and chanterelles

Nuts and seeds (source of protein, source of omega-3)

For example, walnuts, almonds, pecans, Brazil nuts, macadamia, cashew nuts, peanuts (unsalted), pistachios (unsalted), flax and chia seeds, psyllium seeds, sunflower seeds and pine nuts

Herbs and herbs (small nutrient bombs and full of secondary plant substances)

For example, thyme, rosemary, parsley, chervil, coriander, basil, chives, turmeric, ginger and cinnamon

Cereals (high in fibre and protein)

Always go for the wholemeal variety, i.e. wholemeal bread, wholemeal pasta and wholemeal couscous. Bulgur, quinoa, amaranth, wheat germ, kamut, spelt, rye, barley, millet and oat flakes

Bread (high in fibre and protein)

Wholemeal bread, preferably coarse-grained; sourdough bread

Fruit (rich in fibre and colourful due to secondary plant compounds)

Berries of any kind such as blueberries, blackberries, raspberries and strawberries

Apple, pear, plum, peach, apricot—all with skin if possible

Orange, grapefruit, dates, coconut, dried fruits

(Attention: pressed as juice only in small quantities, otherwise there is a lot of fructose.) The rule of thumb is do not juice more fruit than you would normally eat as a whole piece of fruit.

Oil

High-quality cold-pressed olive oil (look for "extra virgin" on the label), rapeseed oil (cold-pressed), linseed oil, pumpkin seed oil

Fish (as rich in fat as possible as a source of omega-3, protein, vitamin D)
For example, salmon, herring, mackerel, trout and sardines

25.5   What You Should Avoid

Sugar: such as industrially produced biscuits, cakes and sweets

Soft drinks of all kinds (very high sugar content)

Ready-made products of any kind: often contain large amounts of hidden sugar and salt

White flour (calorically devoid of nutrients)

Sausage and finished meat products: all industrially produced meat products (sugar and salt content)

All highly heated fatty fried and baked goods: such as French fries, chips, crisps, croissants and other fatty baked goods (keyword: trans-fats)

Milk and dairy products: in moderation at best, because the last word has not yet been spoken here. Which adult animal drinks milk? Milk is a growth drink for newborns—full of protein, fat, sugar in the form of lactose, vitamins and minerals, but it is not a refreshment drink for adults. In adults, growth makes no biological sense and at best increases the risk of cell proliferation and thus possibly also the risk of cancer (Chap. 23, results of The China Study). There is certainly nothing wrong with a glass of milk now and then or a portion with coffee or tea. But here, too, the dose is the poison. Yoghurt, kefir, certain cheeses or quark as so-called fermented milk products—which means predigested by lactic acid bacteria—do not seem to have any adverse effect. If anything, the lactic acid bacteria have a favourable effect on the intestine (keyword: microbiome).

Meat: If meat, then in moderation and from free-range organic grazing animals which have also "eaten well". Make meat a side dish.

25.6   No "Rush Jobs"

A change in diet should be made in stages. The individual steps could, for example, be as described below, but everyone can of course modify them according to their own taste. The important thing is not to take a "rush job" approach.

Success in small steps is the better way.

So: give your body time and drink a lot (unsweetened, of course :-)).
Weeks 1 and 2:

1. Avoid ready-made products.
2. Vegetables as the main food, everything fresh and as seasonal as possible. You can eat as much of them as you want.
3. Add good oils.
4. Supplement vitamin D3 one time a day together with your meal, depending on the season.
5. If you get hungry in between: Take for example, a piece of fruit or a nut mix with you (<u>not</u> if you suffer from nut allergies).
6. Drink plenty of water and/or unsweetened tea.

Weeks 3 and 4:
Everything as above and reduce sugar significantly. No soft drinks!
Sugar withdrawal can cause symptoms such as headaches, fatigue and cravings. Therefore, proceed slowly here, especially if a lot of sugar has been consumed before. Please do not use sweeteners as a substitute!
Weeks 5 and 6:
Everything as above and reduce meat significantly.
Weeks 7 and 8:
Everything as above and significantly reduce white flour products.

25.7   What If …

What if you get hungry in between?
Take a few nuts with you (almonds, walnuts, pecans, etc.—always unsalted) (<u>not</u> if you suffer from nut allergies).
What if the craving for sweets comes?
For example, dark chocolate (90% or more) and dried unsulphured apricots
What if I am thirsty?
Taking in enough fluids is important for the body and also reduces hunger pangs. This of course means unsweetened liquids, such as water, green tea, black tea, filter coffee, ginger water, and lemon or lime water.

What if I do not like fish?

Alternative good sources of omega-3 are nuts, especially walnuts, chia and linseed, as well as linseed and rapeseed oil, but also olive oil or avocadoes are especially good.

25.8   Is There Anything Missing for the Start?

Now you have a list of "goodies" that should be favoured and a list of "baddies" that should be reduced or best avoided altogether. But perhaps you still lack the spark to put these recommendations into practice, what to prepare for breakfast or what to cook for lunch or dinner? In this case, the following selection of recipes is intended as a "small starter set" to make it easier to get started.

> Because as Johann Wolfgang von Goethe said: "It is not enough to know, one must also apply; it is not enough to want, one must also do".

Many of my patients and I have experienced that this change in diet makes us more alert and fit both in mind and body. A positive side effect is that one's body weight probably also normalises naturally.

It is important to point out in any recipe selection that a good recipe stands and falls with the quality of the food that is used. When shopping, it is therefore important to look for good quality. Let's go.

25.9   Recipes to Try Out: The Small "Starter Set"

You will find a small selection of my favourite recipes here. I would be delighted if you like the dishes as much as we do. For further inspiration, I have compiled a few of my favourite cookbooks (see appendix). And another practical tip for those who do not have time to cook at lunchtime—which is probably true for the majority. We have found that cooking larger quantities in the evening also provide for the next day's lunch. And now, have fun and enjoy!

Examples for Breakfast:
Home-made wholemeal bread (30 cm **loaf** tin)

450 g wholemeal flour	into large bowl and mix with
1 tsp salt	and
125 g sunflower seeds	and
100 g pumpkin seeds	and
100 g dried cranberries	and
2 tbsp chia seeds	mix well.
25 g fresh organic yeast	into a second bowl and mix with
425 mL warm water	and
1 tsp agave syrup	and leave to rest for 5 min.

Then combine the yeast mixture with the flour-grain mixture and mix well (with a wooden spoon or your hands).

Place the whole in a lightly oiled baking tin (approx. 30 cm long), cover with a kitchen towel at room temperature and leave to rest for approx. 45 min.

Remove the cloth, preheat the oven and bake at 220 °C convection oven (fan-assisted oven) for 45 min. After approx. 30 min, remove the bread from the baking tin and bake on the rack without the baking tin for the last 15 min.

Remove the bread, leave to cool and enjoy.

Nuts and seeds bread (30 cm loaf tin)

100 g sunflower seeds	and
100 g pumpkin seeds	and
135 g linseed	and
100 g pine nuts (alternatively almonds, walnuts, pecans)	and
220 g millet flakes	and
3 tablespoons chia seeds	and
6 tbsp psyllium husks	and
1.5 tbsp salt	mix all together in a bowl. In a separate bowl mix
525 mL water	with
1.5 tbsp agave syrup	and
4.5 tbsp or 45 g butter or coconut oil	together. Pour the contents of this mixture over the ingredients in the other bowl and mix everything properly.

Pour everything into the baking tin lined with baking paper, press the mixture down well with a spoon and leave to stand for at least 2 h. Then place the baking tin on the middle shelf in the preheated oven at 175 °C convection oven and bake the bread for 30 min.

Then remove the bread upside down from the baking tin and bake on baking paper for a further 40 min.

Leave the bread to cool, and it can then be wrapped in the baking paper. It stays fresh for a good few days.

Both breads are delicious with a sweet or savoury spread. You can use honey or fresh jam, olive oil with egg or the spreads described below, such as guacamole, bruschetta, hummus or fish paste.

Smoothie with avocado, nuts and berries (serves 2)

1 avocado	Remove from the skin with a spoon and place in the blender.
1 handful green salad (or spinach)	Add
1 handful of mixed nuts	Add
1 handful frozen blueberries	Add
2 tbsp olive oil or linseed oil	Add
1 tsp barley grass	Add
1 tsp wheat germ	Add
1/2 tsp maca powder (optional)	
If necessary, add a little vanilla	Add
	and mix everything at low speed, pour into a glass and enjoy.

Smoothie with avocado, nuts and mango (serves 2)

1 avocado	Remove from the peel and place in the blender.
1 handful green salad (or spinach leaves)	Add
1 handful of mixed nuts	Add
1 handful frozen mango	Add
1 lime	Squeeze and add
2 tbsp olive oil or linseed oil	Add
1 tsp barley grass	Add
1 tsp wheat germ	Add
1/2 tsp maca powder (optional)	
If necessary, add a little vanilla	Add and mix everything at low speed, pour into a glass and enjoy.

Muesli with berries (for 2 people)

6–8 tbsp oat flakes	with
2 tsp chia seeds	and
300 g natural yoghurt	Mix
400 g raspberries (or blueberries)	150 g puree of them and mix. Add to
2 tbsp chopped almonds	and top with
50 g berries	and enjoy.

Quinoa porridge (2 people)

100 g quinoa	Wash well; mix in 150 mL water with
2 tbsp cranberries (dried)	Simmer for 15–20 min. Add
2 tsp cinnamon powder	Season and mix quinoa with
2 teaspoons almond slivers	and top with
100 g blueberries	and enjoy.

Ayurveda porridge with apple walnut topping (serves 2)

70 g gluten-free rolled oats	with
200 mL almond milk	and
200 mL water	bring to the boil once. Reduce heat again and add
1 tsp cinnamon powder	and
1/2 teaspoon ground cardamom	and
2 tablespoons hemp seeds, coarsely ground	and
1/2 teaspoon ground vanilla	and simmer for 2–3 min, stirring for a few minutes
	Remove from the cooker.
	Remove from the heat. Then mix in
2 tsp coconut oil	and cover the mixture
	Cover and leave to infuse for 2 min.

Apple-walnut topping:

2 tablespoons ghee	in water in a saucepan and heat
1–2 apples	Slice and add
1 tsp cinnamon powder	and steam for 10 min until soft.
	Stew
50 g chopped walnuts	Mix in.

Pour the porridge into two bowls and add the topping. Sweeten with maple syrup (alternatively with honey) and enjoy.

Banana pancakes (serves 2)

2 eggs	Whisk
1 banana	Mash and add
1 tablespoon protein powder (vanilla or chocolate)	and mix everything together.
1 tsp of coconut oil	Heat in a frying pan and bake small pancakes.

Top with maple syrup or agave syrup with the strawberries or blueberries and enjoy.

Apple-nut curd (for 2 persons)

400 g curd cheese	with
Apple sauce (amount according to personal taste)	and
2 pinches of vanilla powder	Mix
2 apples	Coarsely grate or grate
4 tbsp sultanas	Add
10 pecans or walnuts	Chop, top and enjoy.

Wholemeal bread (toasted) with avocado, cashew nuts and fried eggs (for 1–2 people)

1 ripe avocado	Halve and scrape out the flesh with a spoon
1 tablespoon olive oil	and
1 tsp lemon juice	and
Sea salt	and
freshly ground pepper	Mix
Chop a small handful of cashew nuts	Add
2 small eggs	Break into the pan with
2 tbsp olive oil (coconut oil also works well)	Fry until the egg white has set and season with a little salt and pepper.
Toast 2 slices of wholemeal bread	
Top with avocado mash, cashew nuts if using and fried eggs, enjoy.	

Cream cheese with herbs, egg and cucumber (for 1–2 people)

2 eggs	Boil for 8 min, rinse and leave to cool.
30 g mixed herbs	Wash, dry, pluck off the leaves and finely chop (basil, cress, parsley, chives)
200 g cottage cheese	with herbs and 1 finely chopped egg
	Mix
2 tsp lemon juice	Add and mix with
Sea salt	and
freshly ground pepper	Season
1 small cucumber	Cut into thin slices.

Spread bread slices with herb-egg-fresh cheese mixture. Place the cucumber and egg slices on top. Season with salt and pepper, top with some herbs and enjoy.

Examples for Lunch and Evening
Tomato soup (serves 4)

600 g fresh tomatoes	Wash, halve and place on a baking tray. On baking paper (cherry, bush, etc.)
4 cloves of peeled garlic	and
2–3 rosemary cloves	and
2–3 thyme sprigs	Place on the tray
2–3 tbsp olive oil	Over
1/2 tsp icing sugar (optional)	Also sprinkle over the top
Freshly ground pepper	Over it
1 teaspoon sea salt	Over the top. Place the tray in a preheated oven at 180 degrees C convection oven for approx. 45 min.
1 white medium onion	Coarsely chop and cut into pieces.
1–2 tbsp olive oil	In a soup pot and sauté.
Remove the rosemary and thyme sprigs from the baked tomato mixture, and then add the mixture to the soup pot and stir.	
800 mL–1 L vegetable stock	Add the vegetable stock; simmer for max. 10 min over medium heat.
Chop 1 handful of fresh basil leaves	and mix into the soup. Leave to cool.
Then put the soup into the blender and blend to a fine consistency.	
Season with fresh pepper and sea salt to taste. Serve in a soup plate and enjoy.	

Courgette soup with mint and feta (serves 4)

4–5 medium courgettes	Cut into slices, add
4 whole peeled garlic cloves	
2 tablespoons olive oil	Sweat for 5–10 min. Then pour
approx. 750 mL vegetable stock	over it, enough to cover the courgettes. Simmer for 5–10 min.
Chop 2 tbsp. fresh mint leaves	and add to the soup.
80 g feta	Stir into the soup.
Remove the soup from the heat, allow to cool slightly, then transfer to a blender and blend until a fine consistency is achieved.	
Add salt and fresh black pepper to taste. Pour the soup into the plates and top with a few mint leaves and some feta crumbs and enjoy.	

Cauliflower soup with fried mushrooms and roasted pumpkin seeds (serves approx. 4)

500–600 g cauliflower	Cut into florets
1 onion	Dice
1 tsp coconut oil	Heat in a frying pan, add the onion and fry until golden brown; add the cauliflower and fry for another 2–3 min. Add

500 mL vegetable stock	Deglaze and continue to simmer, approx. 15 min, until the cauliflower is well done, then puree and
2 tbsp lemon juice	Add to the puree
1 large tbsp cashew puree	Also add and mix with
1/2 tsp honey	Season to taste,
A little nutmeg freshly grated to taste	
Sea salt	Season to taste,
Freshly grated pepper	Season to taste.
1 small handful of pumpkin seeds	Heat in a pan and gently roast pumpkin seeds for 3–5 min. Then refrigerate.
3–4 mushrooms	Cut into slices; heat oil in a frying pan, fry mushrooms and season with salt and pepper.
1/2 bunch of parsley	Chop

Divide the soup between the plates and top with pumpkin seeds, mushrooms and parsley and enjoy.

Carrot soup with ginger and orange (serves approx. 4)

8–10 medium carrots	Peel and dice.
2 garlic cloves	Peel and dice.
1–2 shallots	Peel and dice.
Ginger 2–3 cm piece	Peel and dice.
1 tsp coconut oil	Heat in a pan and fry all the cubes in it for 5–10 min until lightly browned and then browned and then mix with
250 mL coconut milk	and
500 mL vegetable stock	Deglaze and simmer for approx. 15 min.
2 oranges	Freshly squeeze and add the juice. Blend everything with a hand blender until creamy and add the
Sea salt	and
Cayenne pepper	Season to taste.
1/2 bunch of parsley	Chop
Alternatively, coriander	

Divide the soup between plates and top with coriander or parsley and enjoy.

Wholemeal spaghetti with avocado basil pesto and fried salmon cubes (serves 4)

Wash four salmon fillets (wild salmon is best), dab dry, dice and marinate with

1 pinch of sea salt	and
1/2 tsp pepper	and
Some chilli flakes (optional)	and add
Juice of 3 organic limes	
	When marinated, set aside.
1 handful of pine nuts	Roast without oil over low heat.
2 ripe avocados	Remove the flesh and dice.
1 bunch of basil	Wash, dry and cut into very small pieces.
Puree the chopped basil, remaining lime juice, toasted pine nuts and avocado in a blender and add to the mixture.	
Salt, pepper	and with
1/2 tsp honey	Season to taste.
200–240 g wholemeal spaghetti	Cook according to package instructions.
Rapeseed oil	Heat in a pan and fry the marinated salmon in it.

Mix the pasta with the pesto (basil/pine/avocado mix) in a pan (if necessary, add a little pasta water until it has a creamy consistency) and top with sautéed salmon cubes and enjoy.

Asian vegetable pan with wholemeal rice (serves 4)

2 carrots	and
1 handful of broccoli florets	and
1 pack of sugar snap peas	and
6 mushrooms	and
1 red pepper	and
1 yellow pepper	and
1/2 courgette	and
1–2 cloves of garlic	and
2 handfuls of bean sprouts	and
3 cm piece of fresh ginger	and
1 handful of unsalted peanuts (not in the case of a nut allergy)	and/or
Cashew nuts	Wash vegetables and cut into small pieces. Broccoli into very small florets
2 tsp rapeseed oil	Heat pan with rapeseed oil; put vegetables, garlic, mushrooms, nuts and sprouts; and sauté until crisp with
Vegetable stock	and
Soy sauce	and deglaze with
Salt, pepper	and
2 tsp sesame seeds	and
Lemon juice	Season to taste.
1 packet wholemeal rice	Cook according to the package instructions.

Serve the rice with the Asian vegetables and enjoy.

Potato-carrot-pumpkin curry with red lentils (serves approx. 6–8)

1 small butternut squash	Dice
6 carrots	Dice
4 medium potatoes	Dice
1 onion	Chop
3–4 fresh garlic cloves	Chop
5 cm fresh ginger	Chop
5–6 tbsp lentils	Wash well.
1 tsp coconut oil	Heat in a frying pan and add all the
chopped and	diced vegetables and the lentils into the pan and sauté.
1 tsp vegetable stock powder	Dissolve with a little hot water.
2–3 tsp curry powder	Add to the pan to deglaze.
250 mL coconut milk	Add and simmer until the vegetables are cooked. If necessary, add a little
water	if too much has evaporated.
Lemon juice	Freshly squeeze and add
Salt and pepper	Add and finally
1–2 tsp honey	Stir in.
Serve in soup plates and enjoy.	

Bean stew with feta (serves 8)

2 red onions	and
2 garlic cloves	Dice
100 g parsley root	and
150 g carrots	Peel and cut into small cubes. Put everything in.
2 tablespoons olive oil	Sauté
Sea salt	Season
600 g tomatoes	Add the chopped tomatoes to the vegetables and steam until soft.
300 g cooked kidney beans	and
300 g white beans	Rinse well and mix with
Paprika powder, sweet	and
Salt and fresh pepper	to taste. From
10 stems of thyme	Strip off the leaves.
400 g feta	Dice.
Top the bean stew with feta and thyme leaves and enjoy.	

Lentils on courgette noodles (serves 4)

100 g brown lentils	Boil in 250 mL water for approx. 20 min until soft.
1 onion	and
1 clove garlic	Finely dice.
100 g celeriac	and

150 g carrots	Peel and dice finely. Dice all in.
2 tablespoons olive oil	Sauté
100 mL red wine	Add and let it boil down for about 10 min. Then
500 g strained tomatoes	Add the tomatoes and continue to simmer for 15 min. Add the lentils and simmer for another 5 min.

For the courgette noodles:

Wash three long thin medium-sized courgettes and cut into spaghetti shapes with a spiral slicer. Cook in the pan with

2 tbsp olive oil	Cook for a few minutes.
100 g Parmesan	Grate

Put the courgette noodles on the plate, top with the lentil-tomato-carrot mixture and enjoy.

Vegetables from the oven with goats' cheese (serves 4)

300 g aubergines	and
300 g courgettes	and
200 g red pepper	and
200 g yellow pepper	Wash, clean and cut into pieces, and mix everything together with
4 sprigs of rosemary	Place on a packing tray.
4 tablespoons olive oil	Pour over it.
Sea salt and fresh pepper	Season and bake at 200 °C in convection oven for approx. 40 min until the vegetables are soft.
4 slices of goats' cheese	Place on top of the vegetables, grill and enjoy.

Cauliflower "steaks" (serves 2–4)

1 cauliflower	Wash well and cut into 3 cm thick slices (steaks).
Olive oil	Brush both sides of the cauliflower well with oil and place on baking paper. Bake in a preheated oven (180 °C in convection oven) for approx. 25–30 min until the steaks are golden brown, turning in between. When golden brown, remove from the oven, then place 1 slice of soft goats' cheese on each "steak" and return to the oven until the cheese has melted.

Remove the cauliflower steaks from the oven, season with salt and pepper and enjoy.

Herb salmon with steamed chard (serves 2)

Wash 2 salmon fillets approx. 150 g (without skin)	Dab dry and season with
Salt	and
Pepper from the mill	Season
2 stalks of parsley	Wash, shake dry, pluck off the leaves and finely chop
2 stalks of chives	Wash, dry and chop. Mix both herbs, cover and set aside.
400 g chard	Clean and wash, and cut the leaves off the stems. Cut the leaves into approx. 1 cm strips, and the stems into 1/2 cm wide strips.
1 shallot	and
1 clove of garlic	Peel and finely dice the garlic.
1 tsp coconut oil	Heat in a pan and steam the salmon fillets on both sides for approx. 8–10 min. Remove from the pan, throw in the chopped herbs and keep warm.
1 tsp rapeseed oil	and
1 tsp butter	In a saucepan, sauté the shallot, garlic and chard stems for 2–3 min. Season with salt and pepper.
100 mL vegetable stock	Bring to the boil, cover and simmer for approx. 5 min. Add the chard leaves and cook for approx. 1 min.

Season the vegetables to taste, arrange on the plates, arrange the salmon fillet on the bed of chard and enjoy.

Beetroot carpaccio (serves 2–4)

2 cooked beetroots	Cut into very thin slices and arrange flat on a plate.
2 tablespoons balsamic vinegar	and
4 tablespoons olive oil	with
salt and pepper	and spread over the beetroot slices. Top with
1 tablespoon crème fraiche	and
1 tbsp chopped walnuts	and
freshly grated horseradish	and enjoy.

Summer salad with watermelon and feta (serves 4)

75 g cashew nuts (optional)	Chop coarsely and roast in a pan without fat. Then immediately place them on a plate.
1/4–1/2 watermelon approx. 500 g	Dice the flesh and place in a bowl.
20–40 g mint leaves	Pluck the leaves from the stems and add the leaves to the melon.
250 g feta	Dice or crumble and add to the mixture.

2 tablespoons white acetone balsamic vinegar	with
juice of 1 lime	and
1/2 tsp salt	and
Pepper from the mill	and
3 tbsp olive oil	to a dressing and mix into the salad.
Top with the roasted cashews (if using) and enjoy.	

Pear rocket and parmesan salad (serves 4)

3 pears	Cut the pears into slices and gently fry them in a pan over a moderate heat with a spoon of organic butter.
2 tablespoons olive oil	Fry
Salt and pepper	Add
400 g rocket salad	Wash, dab dry and spread on a plate, then place the pear slices on top and sprinkle with freshly grated Parmesan and enjoy.

Hummus

Chickpeas (1 small tin)	Rinse in a colander with water and drain. Mix with
Salt	and
1 tsp cumin	in a blender on low speed.
Juice of 1 lemon	and
3–4 basil leaves	Add
50 mL olive oil	Slowly drizzle in the olive oil. Blend on low speed until a coarse paste and mix with
Salt	and
Pepper from the mill	Season to taste. Serve in a bowl and enjoy on bread, for example.

Guacamole

2 avocados	Peel with a spoon, pit and mash in a bowl. Mix with the juice of one lime drizzle.
1 handful of cherry tomatoes	Cut into quarters or smaller and
1 medium shallot	Chop
1 small clove of garlic	Mix with the avocado.
1–2 tbsp olive oil	Add and mix with
Salt	and
Pepper from the mill	Season to taste; garnish with parsley if desired and enjoy.

Bruschetta with olive oil

1 ciabatta	Cut into slices
2 cloves of garlic	Rub the bread with the cut surface.
4 tbsp olive oil	Slowly in a frying pan, add the slices of bread and toast until golden brown.
400 g cocktail tomatoes	Finely dice.
1/2 bunch of basil	Wash and cut into fine strips.
1 small clove of garlic	Finely chop and add (can also be omitted as desired).
5 tbsp olive oil	Add and
1/2 tsp salt	and
Pepper from the mill	Mix everything together. Place the bread on the plate while it is still warm and top with the tomato mixture.
	Top with the remaining basil and enjoy.

Tuna paste

1 can of tuna (150 g)	together with
1 tsp capers	and
1 cup cream cheese	into a bowl.
1 small shallot	Chop
Chop the fresh herbs (parsley, thyme).	
1/2 clove of garlic	Peel off the skin and chop.
Add a little lemon juice	and puree everything together.
Spread the paste on fresh bread	and enjoy.

Avocado sandwich

1 slice of wholemeal bread	with a previously mashed
Avocado	
Cucumber slices	Cut into thin slices and place on top of the avocado and top with radish slices and sprouts.
	Enjoy.

Salmon hummus sandwich

1 slice of wholemeal bread	with
hummus (see above for recipe)	spread
(Smoked) salmon slice	on top and cover with
Lemon juice	drizzle. Top with
Avocado slices	and
Cress	drape and decorate with
Sea Salt	and
Pepper from the mill	Season to taste and enjoy.

Bruschetta fried egg sandwich

1 slice of wholemeal bread	with
Bruschetta (see above for recipe)	Top
Fry 1 egg	and place on the bruschetta and sprinkle with
Sea salt	and
Pepper from the mill	Season to taste and enjoy.

An interesting variation instead of a slice of bread:

You can toast a thick slice (approx. 1 cm) of a large sweet potato in the toaster several times until it is crispy on the outside and soft on the inside or bake it in a preheated oven at 180 degrees for approx. 20 min. Then place the sandwich ingredients on top and enjoy like a sandwich.

Kale chips to "nibble" in the evening—the healthy alternative to crisps

Curly kale	Cut off the stems, wash well and dry very well.
	Cut into approx. 5–8 cm pieces. Place in a bowl.
	Add olive oil enough so that the kale leaves can be massaged in well with the oil all the way to the ends.
1–2 pinches of sea salt	Mix well and spread on an oven tray lined with baking paper.
Bake in a preheated oven at 180 degrees for about 10 min until the kale leaves are crispy. Check regularly, as every oven is different, and the kale leaves can burn easily.	
Put everything in a bowl and enjoy.	
Important: If the kale leaves have not been patted dry properly at the beginning, they will remain limp even during baking!	

<u>For the hunger pangs in between meals:</u>

– Nut mixture always with you (as stated above, **not** if you are allergic to nuts)
– Dried, unsulphured apricots
– Dark chocolate with more than 90% cocoa
– One piece of fresh fruit

And now **enjoy!**

26

The Most Important Recommendations Summarised

26.1 Nutritional Optimisation

As far as possible, convenience products should be avoided and the diet should be optimised step by step towards "real food", i.e. unprocessed food. A plant-based, fibre-rich diet with good oils is recommended. High salt and sugar consumption should be avoided. If meat consumption cannot be avoided, reduce it and look for good organic quality. On the subject of nutrition, I would like to recommend the excellent book by Bas Kast, "The Diet Compass". And if you would like to dive into the topic of the intestine, I highly recommend the book by Giulia Enders, "Gut" (The Inside Story of Our Body's Most Under-Rated Organ), written in a professionally competent and very humorous way. Another excellent book which came out since the original publication of this one in German is "A Healthier Family for Life: Stress-Free Feasts for a Multi-Diet Family" by Donna Crous. A firm favourite of ours!

26.2 Sun and Vitamin D3

Sunbathing is worthwhile from April to October for the body's own vitamin D production. The best time of day for this is midday between 12.00 and 14.00. A sunbathing break for 10–15 min without sunscreen on the face, décolleté and arms is sufficient for vitamin D production; spending longer in the sun leads to sunburn, which should be avoided at all costs. If spending time outdoors is only rarely possible and in our latitudes during the months

A. Friedrich, *The Multiple Sclerosis Companion*,
https://doi.org/10.1007/978-3-662-67540-3_26

of October to April, vitamin D3 intake is recommended so that blood levels of over 30 ng/mL, preferably 60 ng/mL, can be achieved. On the subject of vitamin D and the sun, I can recommend the literature and lectures by Prof. Dr. med. Jörg Spitz.

26.3   Movement and Relaxation

In this guide, I have focused on nutrition and the gut. However, the importance of exercise for physical and mental health should also be remembered. Exercise, if possible, should take place regularly at least 2–3 times a week for at least half an hour. This is possible for almost everyone, on foot, with a walker or even with a rollator at an individual pace. I have told you about Jennifer's bike ride and about MS sufferers from my consultation who run half marathons or marathons. These are extremes that show:

> Nothing is impossible.

However, it is not about maximum performance, but about everyone integrating movement into their lives with joy within the scope of their possibilities. Exercises are also possible in a wheelchair. While sitting, for example, breathing exercises from qi gong or yoga can stimulate the circulation and activate the body.

Alternating tension and relaxation, like yin and yang, is part of the balance of life. There are numerous studies that provide evidence for the value of physical and mental exercise, e.g. through meditation, yoga or qi gong, in MS. Forms of meditation and mindfulness training are becoming increasingly popular in our regions. MBSR, for example, which stands for "mindfulness-based stress reduction", combines several of these aspects. It is a module for cultivating mindfulness that includes various forms of meditation, gentle yoga and modern psychology. Developed 40 years ago by the American Jon Kabat-Zinn, it is now widely used in outpatient and inpatient care for chronically ill patients. His books on meditation and dealing with illness, stress and pain are highly recommended.

26.4   In Conclusion

And now we come to the end. You have received extensive information about multiple sclerosis in this companion. You now know the possible symptoms and the examination methods including MRI and lumbar puncture. You have gained an intensive insight into the immune system and therefore an understanding of the therapy. You have learnt about the different medications, their indications and mode of action on the immune system. You now know which considerations are necessary to plan an individual MS therapy.

You have read about encouraging case studies in Part III of this book and learned that environmental factors influence our gut and its inhabitants. You have received interesting information on the "communication" between the microbiota, the immune system and the central nervous system from many studies, and I am sure we will learn much more about this in the years to come.

In conclusion, I would therefore like to encourage you to also implement lifestyle changes in your everyday life in addition to your specific MS therapy.

I wish you joy and success along your way!

Glossary

Antigen-presenting cell (APC) It presents the antigen and thereby activates the acquired immune system of T and B lymphocytes with antibody formation.

Autoimmune disease Disease in which the body's own defence—the immune system—reacts and fights against substances that belong to its own body. In the case of MS, the myelin.

Axon Nerve branch via which information is conducted away from the nerve cell ("departure").

Blood–brain barrier (BBB) "Barrier" made up of certain cells that only allow certain particles to pass into the CNS and not others—damaged in MS.

Blue Zones Areas where people are much less likely to live with chronic diseases, grow particularly old and often remain mentally active and physically healthy into old age.

Brain atrophy Decrease in brain tissue due to cell death and, as a result, "reduction" of the total brain volume.

Calcidiol Storage form of vitamin D.

Calcitriol "Armed" vitamin D.

Central nervous system CNS, for short, is made up of the brain and spinal cord and is, so to speak, the "control centre" and "nerve highway" of the body.

The China Study Huge, epidemiological nutrition study that looks more closely at the links between food and health/disease.

Cortisone Treatment for acute relapses of MS; helps to reduce the inflammatory response.

CSF Nerve fluid that washes around the brain and spinal cord.

A. Friedrich, *The Multiple Sclerosis Companion*, https://doi.org/10.1007/978-3-662-67540-3

Course-modifying therapy strategy Therapy strategy in which the therapy decision is prognosis-based. The doctor tries to assess the aggressiveness of the course of the disease from the outset on the basis of certain risk factors in order to be able to treat it more individually.

Dendrite Nerve branch via which information is transmitted to the nerve cell ("arrival").

Dendritic cell (DC) Also belongs to the antigen-presenting cells (APCs). Their main task is also the recognition of an intruder and the antigen presentation of foreign cell structures on their cell surface.

Disability progression Progressive pathological and permanent physical impairment due to MS.

Disease-modifying drug (DMD) Medicines used in the course-modifying therapy

Dysbiosis Disturbance of the balance of intestinal microbiotics

EDSS score For expanded disability status scale; a scale that provides information about the degree of disability of a person with MS.

Environmental factors Those factors that affect the individual from the outside and can also have a changing effect.

Eubiosis Presence of a stable, balanced, species-rich gut microbiota.

Experimental autoimmune encephalomyelitis (EAE) Experimentally induced MS-like disease in the mouse.

Fatigue Extreme fatigue, which can occur as a symptom of MS disease.

Faecal microbiota transplantation (FMT) Stool transplant.

German Multiple Sclerosis and Fertility Registry (DMSKW) and the UK MS Pregnancy Register Pregnancy registers, which collect the essential facts on pregnancy/breastfeeding and MS.

Granulocyte Part of the innate immune system, fends off infections caused by bacteria, viruses, fungi or parasites.

Gut-associated lymphoid tissue (GALT) Intestinal immune system residing in the intestinal wall.

Gut microbiome Totality of all genes of the microorganisms that populate the intestine.

Gut microbiotics The totality of all microorganisms that colonise the intestine.

Immunoadsorption Proteins (namely immunoglobulins) are (specifically) withdrawn from the body via an access into the vein.

Immunoglobulins Also called antibodies, they are proteins and serve the body's precise defence.

Immunomodulatory, course-modifying therapy Therapy designed to positively influence the chronic course of the disease.

Isoelectric focusing Comparison of serum and cerebrospinal fluid to detect immunoglobulins (IgG) produced in the CNS.

Leukocytes White blood cells (granulocytes, monocytes, lymphocytes).

Lumbar puncture (LP) The extraction of neural fluid.

Lymphatic progenitor cell This gives rise to the lymphocytes in the bone marrow as defence cells.

Magnetic resonance imaging (MRI) Also called magnetic resonance imaging; imaging examination in which individual organs can be examined in different planes and displayed in layers.

Macrophages The "large phagocytes" serve for defence and antigen presentation.

Monocytes Belong to the leukocytes and, like granulocytes, fight off infections. They can migrate from the blood into the tissue and transform into macrophages.

Myelin Sheathing of the nerve fibres; the insulation, so to speak, of the cable that conducts the impulses.

Myeloid progenitor cell This gives rise to the granulocytes and monocytes in the bone marrow.

Next-generation sequencing (NGS) Method to be able to determine the gut microbiota via its genes.

No evidence of disease activity (NEDA) Therapeutic goal in MS therapy; as far as possible no evidence of disease activity.

Oligodendrocyte They form the myelin and wrap the axons with it.

Oligoclonal bands (OCBs) Formed from IgG during examination by isoelectric focusing.

Plasmapheresis Proteins are (non-specifically) removed from the body via an access point in the vein.

Primary progressive MS (PPMS) Primary progressive form of MS (form of progression without the occurrence of relapses).

Reiber diagram Diagram to assess blood–brain barrier function and possible intrathecal immunoglobulin production in the cerebrospinal fluid.

Relapsing-remitting MS (RRMS) Relapsing-remitting form of MS (one relapse is initially followed by a regression until the next relapse).

Secondary progressive MS (SPMS) Secondary progressive form of MS (relapse is not followed by complete remission, disability persists and/or worsens slowly).

Thrust therapy Acute treatment given during MS relapse.

Thymus Gland located behind the breastbone in which the lymphocytes are imprinted. In the course of life, it slowly regresses.

Vitamin D The precursor of a hormone that influences numerous metabolic processes and is important for bone metabolism and also for the immune system.

Western diet Today's predominant diet of the Western world with many convenience foods often with high hidden sugar and salt content, hydrogenated fats, preservatives, emulsifiers and flavour enhancers.

Bibliography

Adorini L, Penna G. Dendritic cell tolerogenicity: a key mechanism in immuno-modulation by vitamin D receptor agonists. Hum Immunol. 2009;70(5):345–52.

Alang N, Kelly CR. Weight gain after fecal microbiota transplanation. Open Forum Infect Dis. 2015;2(1):ofv 004.

Allen AC, Kelly S, Basdeo SA, et al. A pilot study of immunological effects of high dose vitamin D in healthy volunteers. Mult Scler. 2012;18(12):1797–180.

Alrouji M, Manouchehrinia A, Gran B, Constantinescu CS. Effects of cigarette smoke on immunity, neuroinflammation and multiple sclerosis. J Neuroimmunol. 2019:24–34.

Amato MP, et al. Environmental modifiable risk factors for multiple sclerosis: Report from the 2016 ECTRIMS focused workshop. Mult Scler. 2018;24(5):590–603.

Anonymous. Atlas multiple sclerosis resources in the world; 2008. ISBN: 978-92-4-156375-8

Anonymous. https//gesundheitswelt.allianz.de/gesundheit-ernaehrung/abnehmen-diaet/infografik-zucker-in-zahlen.html; n.d.

Arrambide G, Tintore M, Espejo C, et al. The value of oligoclonal bands in the multiple sclerosis diagnostic criteria. Brain. 2018;141:1075–84.

Ascherio A, Mangel KL. Epidemiology of multiple sclerosis: from risk factors to prevention-an update. Seminary's Neurol. 2016;36(2):103–14.

Ascherio, et al. Trans fatty acids and Coronary heart disease. N Eng J Med. 1999;340:1994–8.

Ashtari F, Toghianifar N, Zarkesh-Esfahani SH, Mansourian M. Short-term effect of high dose vitamin D on the level of interleukin 10 in patients with multiple sclerosis: a randomized, double-blind, placebo-controlled clinical trial. Neuroimmunomodulation. 2015;22(6):400–4.

© The Editor(s) (if applicable) and The Author(s), under exclusive license to Springer-Verlag GmbH, DE, part of Springer Nature 2023
A. Friedrich, *The Multiple Sclerosis Companion*, https://doi.org/10.1007/978-3-662-67540-3

Atlas. 2008. Atlas Multiple Sclerosis Resources in the World.

Atlas Multiple Sclerosis Resources in the World 2008; ISBN 978 92 4 156375

Ausgabe D. China Study: Die wissenschaftliche Begründung für eine vegane Ernährungsweise. Verlag systematische Medizin; n.d. isbn:978-3-86401-001-9.

Bäärnhielm M, Hedström AK, Kockum I, et al. Sunlight is associated with decreased multiple sclerosis risk: no interaction with human leucocyte antigen-DRB1*15. Eur J Neurol. 2012;19(7):955–62.

Bäckhed F, Ley RE, Sonnenburg JL, et al. Host-bacterial mutualism in the human intestine. Science. 2005;307:1915–20.

Bäckhed F, Roswall J, Peng Y, et al. Dynamics and stabilization of the human gut microbiome during the first year of life. Cell Host Microbe. 2015;17(5):690–703.

Bang C, Weidenbach K, Gutsmann T, Heine H, Schmitz RA. The intestinal archaea Methanosphaera stadtmanae and Methanobrevibacter smithii activate human dentritic cells. PLoS One. 2014;9:e99411.

Barragan M, Good M, et al. Regulation of dendritic cell function by vitamin D. Nutrients. 2015;7(9):8127–51.

Berer K, Mues M, Koutrolos M, et al. Commensal microbiota and myelin autoantigen cooperate to trigger autoimmune demyelination. Nature. 2011;479:538–41.

Berer K, Gerdes LA, Cekanaviciute E, Jia X, Xiao L, Xia Z, Liu C, Klotz L, Stauffer U, Baranzini SE, Kümpfel T, Hohfeld R, Krishnamoorthy G, Wekerle H. Gut microbiota from multiple sclerosis patients enables spontaneous autoimmune encephalomyelitis in mice. PNAS. 2017;114(40):10,719–24.

Buchter B, Dunkel M, Li J. Multiple sclerosis: a disease of affluence? Neuroepidemiology. 2012;39(1):51–6.

Buettner D, Skemp S. Blue Zones: Lessons from the worlds longest lived. Am J Lifestyle Med. 2016;10(5):318–21.

Buscarinu MC, Cerasoli B, Annibali V, et al. Altered intestinal permeability in patients with relapsing-remitting multiple sclerosis: a pilot study. Mult Scler. 2017;23(3):442–6.

Buscarinu MC, Romano S, Mechelli R, et al. Intestinal Permeability in relapsing-remitting multiple sclerosis. Neurotherapeutics. 2018;15(1):68–74.

Calabrese P, Penner IK. Cognitive dysfunctions in multiple sclerosis-a "multiple disconnection syndrome"? J Neurol. 2007;254(2):II18–21.

Campbell TC, Campbell TM. The China Study: the most comprehensive study of nutrition ever conducted and the startling implications for diet, weight loss and long term health. Ney York: Benbella Books; 2006; ISBN 978-1-932100-66-2

Chen J, Chia N, Kalari KR, et al. Multiple sclerosis patients have a distinct gut microbiota compared to healthy controls. Sci Rep. 2016;6:28,484.

Clemente JC et al. The microbiome of uncontacted Amerindians. Sci Adv 2015; 1(3). pii:e1500183

Collins SM, Bercik P. The relationship between intestinal microbiota and the central nervous system in normal gastrointestinal function and disease. Gastroenterology. 2009;136:2003–14.

Colpitts SL, Kasper EJ, et al. A bidirectional association between the gut microbiota and CNS disease in a biphasic murine model of multiple sclerosis. Gut Microbes. 2017:1–13.

Crous D. A healthier family for life: stress-free feasts for a multi-diet family; n.d. isbn:978-1-4721-4411-9.

Das MS-Register. MSFP: MS Forschungs- und Projektentwicklungs-gGmbH. http:// www.dmsg.de/multiple-sklerose-news/ms-forschung. Accessed 6 Feb 2019.

David LA, Maurice CF, Carmody RN, et al. Diet rapidly and reproducibly alters the human gut microbiome. Nature. 2014;505:559–63.

De Paepe M, Leclerc M, Tinsley CR, et al. Bacteriophages: an underestimated role in human and animal health? Front Cell Infect Microbiol. 2014;4:39.

Dendrou CA, Fugger L. Immunomodulation in multiple sclerosis: promises and pitfalls. Curr Option Immunol. 2017;49:37–43.

Deutschen Gesellschaft für Neurologie. Empfehlungen der Deutschen Gesellschaft für Neurologie (DGN) in der Therapie der MS. 2023.

Die ErnährungsDocs. ZS Verlag; n.d. isbn:978-3-89883-561-9.

Dörr J, Ohlraun S, Skarabis H, Paul F. Efficacy of Vitamin D supplementation in multiple sclerosis (EVIDIMS Trial): study protocol for a randomized controlled trial. Trials. 2012;13:15.

Dörr J, Bäcker-Koduah P, et al. High-dose vitamin D supplementation in multiple sclerosis—results from the randomized EVIDIMS trial. Mult Scler J Exp Trans Clin. 2020;6(1)

Duncan SH, Holtrop G, Lobley GE, Calder AG, Stewaert CS, Flint HJ. Contribution of acetate to butyrate formation by human faecal bacteria. Br J Nutr. 2004;91:915–23.

Ebers GC, Sadovnick AD, Risch NJ. A genetic basis for familial aggregation in multiple sclerosis. Canadian Collaborative Study Group. Nature. 1995;377:150–1.

Elias-Hamp B, et al. Wenn Frauen mit Multiple Sklerose sich Kinder wünschen. Thieme Praxis Report. 2020:1–16.

Enders G. Gut: the inside story of our body's most under-rated organ; n.d. isbn:9781911344773.

Esselstyn CB, Ellis SG, Medendorp SV, Crowe TD. A strategy to arrest and reserve coronary artery disease: a 5-year longitudinal study of a single physician's practice. J Fam Pract. 1995;41:560–8.

Ferreira GB, Vanherwegen AS, et al. Vitamin D3 induces tolerance in human dendritic cells by activation of intracellular metabolic pathways. Cell Rep. 2015;10(5):711–25.

fit mit fett, Die Omega-3-Revolution, Dr. Ulrich Strunz, Andreas Kopp; Heyne Verlag; n.d.

Galli C. Antiatherogenic components of olive oil. Curr Artheroscler Rep. 2001;3(1):64–70.

Gerard PH. Spektrum der Wissenschaft; Spezial: Biologie-Medizin-Hirnforschung 1/16. Gesunde Ernährung. n.d.; www.spektrum.de/artikel/1382042

Giovannoni G, Tomic D, Bright JR, et al. No evident disease activity: the use of combined assessments in the management of patients with multiple sclerosis. Mult Scler. 2017;23(9):1179–87.

Goodin DS. The genetic and environmental bases of complex human-disease: extending the utility of twin-studies. PloS One. 2012;7(12):e47875.

Goodin DS. The nature of genetic susceptibility to multiple sclerosis: constraining the possibilities. BMC Neurol. 2016;16:56.

Gorham ED, Garland CF, et al. Optimal vitamin D status for colorectal cancer prevention: a quantitative meta analysis. Am J Prev Med. 2007;32(3):210–6.

Haghikia A, Linker R. Diät, Mikrobiom und Multiple Sklerose. Akt Neurol. 2018;45:24–8.

Haghikia A, Jörg ST, Duscha A, et al. Dietary fatty acids directly impact central nervous system autoimmunity via the small intestine. Immunity. 2015;43:818–29.

Hansen CP, Overvad K, Kyro C, Olsen A, Tjonneland A, Johnsen SP, et al. Adherence to a healthy Nordic diet and risk of stroke: a Danish cohort study. Strike. 2017;48:259–64.

Hart PH, Gorman S. Exposure to UV wave-lengths in sunlight suppresses immunity: to what extent is UV-induced vitamin D3 the mediator responsible? Clin Biochem Rev. 2013;34(1):3–13.

Hathcock JN, Shao A, Vieth R, Heaney R. Risk assessment for vitamin D. Am J Clin Nutr. 2007;85(1):6–18.

Health Care Atlas of the Central Institute. 2023. Versorgungsatlas des Zentralinstituts für Kassenärztliche Versorgung.

Hedström AK, Olsson T, Alfredsson L. Body mass index during adolescence, rather than childhood, is critical in determining MS risk. MultScler. 2016;22(7):878–83.

Helander HF, Fändriks L. Surface area of the digestive tract-revisited. Scan J Gastroenterol. 2014;49(6):681–9.

Hellwig K, Wilkening W. Kinderwunsch bei Multipler Sklerose. Nervenheilkunde. 2020;39:141–6.

Holick MF. Environmental factors that influence the cutaneous production of vitamin D. Am J Clin Nutr Band. 1995;61(3):638–45.

Howell OW, Reeves CA, Nicholas R, et al. Meningeal inflammation is widespread and linked to cortical pathology in multiple sclerosis. Brain. 2011;134:2755–71.

Hucke S, Wiendl H, Klotz L. Implications of dietry salt intake for multiple sclerosis pathogenesis. Mult Scler J. 2016;22(2):133–9.

Ivanov II, Atarashi K, Manel N, et al. Induction of intestinal Th17 cells by segmented filamentous bacteria. Cell. 2009;139(3):485–98.

Jangi S, Gandhi R, Cox LM, Li N, von Glehn F, et al. Alterations of human gut microbiome in multiple sclerosis. Nat Commun. 2016;7:12,015.

Jellinek G. Multiple Sklerose überwinden. Narayana Verlag; 2018a. p. 120–3. ISBN: 978-3-946566-98-4

Jellinek G. Overcoming multiple sclerosis, deutsche Übersetzung Multiple Sklerose überwinden. Narayana Verlag; 2018c. p. 119–52. ISBN: 978-3-946566-98-4

Jenkins DJ, Kendall CW, Marchie A, Faulkner DA, Wong JM, de Souza R, Emam A, Parker TL, Vidgen E, Lapsley KG, Trautwein EA, Josse RG, Leiter LA, Conelly PW. Effects of a dietary portfolio of cholesterol-lowering foods vs lovastatin on serum lipids and C-reactive protein. JAMA. 2003;290(4):502–10.

Jörg S, Grohme DA, Erzler M, Binsfeld M, Haghikia A, Müller DN, Linker RA, Kleinewietfeld M. Environmental factors in autoimmune diseases and their role in multiple sclerosis. Cell Mol Life Sci. 2016;73:4611–22.

Joshi S, Pantalena LC, Lui XK, et al. 1,25-Dihydroxyvitamin D3 ameliorates Th17 autoimmunity via transcriptional modulation of interleukin-17A. Mol Cell Biol. 2011;31:3653–69.

Kabat-Zinn J. Mindfulness for beginners: reclaiming the present moment—and your life; n.d. isbn:9781604076585.

Kahleova H, Matoulek M, Malinska H, Oliyarnik O, Kazdova L, Neskudla T, Skoch A, Hajek M, Hill M, Kahle M, Pelikanova T. Vegetarian diet improves insulin resistance and oxidative stress markers more than conventional diet in subjects with Type 2 diabetes. Diabet Med. 2011;28(5):549–59.

Kast B. Der Ernährungskompass, Das Kochbuch, C. Bertelsmann; n.d.-a ISBN: 978-3-570-10381-4.

Kast B. The diet compass: the 12-step guide to science-based nutrition for a healthier and longer life; n.d.-b. isbn:9781912854936.

Kilsdonk ID, Jonkman LE, Klaver R, et al. Increased cortical grey matter lesion detection in multiple sclerosis with 7 T MRI: a post-mortem verification study. Brain. 2016;139(5):1472–81.

Kiss the Cook. Laura Koerver, Gräfe und Unzer; n.d. ISBN: 978-3-8338-6332-5.

KKNMS (Krankheitsbezogenes Kompetenznetz Multiple Sklerose e.V.) Qualitätshandbuch MS/NMOSD, Ausgabe 2019

Kleinschnitz C, Doerck S. Diagnose, therapie and Risikomanagement der PML bei Multipler Sklerose. DNP. 2013;14:64–9.

Kompetenznetz Multiple Sklerose. Empfehlungen des Krankheitsbezogenen Kompetenznetz Multiple Sklerose (KKNMS). 2021.

Kurtzke JF. Rating neurologic impairment in multiple sclerosis: an expanded disability scale. Neurology. 1983;33(11):1444–52.

Lemberg U. Untersuchung zur Epidemiologie und Therapie des Vitamin D Mangels in Deutschland (Dissertation). Klinik für Nuklearemedizin: Mainz Johannes Gutenberg Universität; 2012.

Levinthal DJ, Rahman A, et al. Adding to the burden: gastrointestinal symptoms and syndromes in multiple sclerosis. Mult Scler Int. 2013:319201.

Linker R, Haghikia A. Rolle des Darmes bei der Multiplen Sklerose. Nervenheilkunde. 2020;39:42–6.

Linker R, Mäurer M. Welche Rolle spielt die Ernährung für die Multiple Sklerose? DNP. 2017;18(S1)

Lucas RM, Ponsonby AL, Dear K, et al. Sun exposure and vitamin D are independent risk factors for CNS demyelination. Neurology. 2011;76:540–8.

Magliozzi R, Howell O, Vora A, Serafini B, Nicholas R, Puopolo M, Reynolds R, Aloisi F. Meningeal B-cell follicles in secondary progressive multiple sclerosis associate with early onset of disease und severe cortical pathology. Brain. 2007;130(4):1089–104.

Major EO, et al. Pathogenesis of progressive multifocal leukoencephalopathy and risks associated with treatments for multiple sclerosis: a decade of lessons learned. Lancet Neurol. 2018;17:467–80.

Martinez-Gonzales MA, Ros E, Estruch R. Primary prevention of cardiovascular disease with a Mediterranean diet supplemented with extra-virgin olive oil or nuts. N Engl J Med. 2018;379(14):1388–9.

Mayer EA, Tillisch K, Gupta A. Gut/brain axis and microbiota. J Clin Invest. 2015;125:926–38.

Montalban X, Gold R, Thompson AJ, et al. ECTRIMS/EAN guideline on the pharmacological treatment of people with multiple sclerosis. Eur J Neurol. 2018;25(2):215–37.

Müller T. Warum es heute so viele MS-Kranke gibt. Ärztezeitung Online. 2018;26:03.

Munger KL, Zhang SM, O'Reilly E, et al. Vitamin D intake and incidence of multiple sclerosis. Neurologie. 2004;62:60–5.

Munger KL, Levin LI, Hollis BW, Howard NS, Ascherio A. Serum 25-hydroxyvitamin D levels and risk of multiple sclerosis. JAMA. 2006;296(23):2832–8.

Munger KL, Chitnis T, Ascherio A. Body size and risk of MS in two cohorts of US women. Neurology. 2009;73(19):1543–50.

O'Hara AM, Shanahan F. The gut flora as a forgotten organ. EMBO Rep. 2006;7:688–93.

Ochoa-Reparaz J, Mielcarz DW, Ditrio LE, et al. Role of gut commensal microflora in the development of experimental autoimmune encephalomyelitis. J Immunol. 2009;183:6041–50.

Oomen CM, et al. Association between trans fatty acid intake and 10 year risk of coronary heart disease in the Zutphen Elderly Study: a prospective population-based study. Lancet. 2001;357:746–51.

Ornish D, Brown SE, Scherwitz LW, et al. Can lifestyle changes reverse coronary heart disease? The Lifestyle Heart Trial. Lancet. 1990;336:129–33.

Penner I-K. Kognitives Screening: Kognition und MS-ein unterschätzen Problem. DNP Der Neurologe und Psychiater 2017a; 18(S1)

Penner I-K. Multiple Sklerose: Kognitive Defizite haben hohe Relevanz für den Alltag. Perspektiven der Neurologie Dtsch Arztbl. 2017b;114(37):12–5.

Polman CH, Reingold SC, Banwell B, et al. Diagnostic criteria for multiple sclerosis: 2010 Revisions to the McDonald criteria. Ann Neurol. 2011;69(2):292–302.

Qin J, et al. A human gut microbial gene catalogue established by metagenomic sequencing. Nature. 2010;464(7285):59–65.

Rabenberg M, Mensink GBM. Vitamin D status in Deutschland. J Health Monitoring. 2016;1(2):36–42.

Ramanujam R, Hedström AK, Manouchehrinia A, Alfredsson L, Olsson T, Bottai M, Hillert J. Effect of smoking cessation on multiple sclerosis prognosis. JAMA Neurol. 2015;72(10):1117–23.

Reiber H. The hyperbolic function: a mathematical solution of the protein flux/CSF flow model for blood–CSF barrier function. J Neurol Sci. 1994;126:240–2.

Richard JL, Yap YA, et al. Dietary metabolites and the gut microbiota: an alternative approach to control inflammatory and autoimmune diseases. Clin Trans Immunol. 2016;5(5):e82.

Ridaura VK, Faith JJ, Rey FE, et al. Gut microbiota from twins discordant for obesity modulate metabolism in mice. Science. 2013;341:S.1079.

Rogers KA, MacDonald M. Therapeutic yoga: symptom management for multiple sclerosis. J Altern Complement Med. 2015;21(11):655–9.

Rotstein D, Montalban X. Reaching an evidence-based prognosis for personalized treatment of multiple sclerosis. Nat Rev Neurol. 2019;15(5):287–300.

Rovira A. When and how to use gadolinium? In: Oral presentation at the 35th European Committee for Treatment and Research in Multiple Sclerosis Congress in Stockholm, Sweden; 11. September 2019. 2019.

Sander C, Voelter HU, et al. Diagnostik der Fatigue bei Multiple Sklerose. Akt Neurol. 2017;44:252–9.

Schiller S, et al. Was bei der pädiatrischen Multiplen Sklerose zu beachten ist. DNP Der Neurol Psychiater; 2016.

Schuhmacher AM, Mahler C, Kerschensteiner M. Pathologie und Pathogenese der progredienten Multiplen Sklerose: Konzepte und Kontroversen. Akt Neurol. 2017;44:476–88.

Serafini B, Rosicarelli B, Magliozzi R, Stigliano E, Alois F. Detection of ectopic B-cell follicles with germinal centers in the meninges of patients with secondary progressive multiple sclerosis. Brain Pathol. 2004;14(2):164–74.

Setzer M. Meditation, Mäuse und Myelin. Nervenheilkunde. 2018;37:745–8.

Siglienti I, Gold R. Therapie der Multiplen Sklerose. Therapietabellen. 2018;7:79.

Simon B, Schmidt S, Lukas C, et al. Improved in vivo detection of cortical lesions in multiple sclerosis using double inversion recovery MR imaging at 3 Tesla. Eur Radiol. 2010;20(7):1675–83.

Sofi F, Cesari F, Abbate R, Gensini GF, Casini A. Adherence to Mediterranean diet and health status: metaanalysis. BMJ. 2008;337:a1344.

Song M, Fung TT, Hu FB, Willett WC, Longo VD, Chan AT, Giovannucci EL. Association of animal and plant protein intake with all-cause and cause-specific mortality. JAMA Intern Med. 2016;176(10):1453–63.

Spitz J, Vitamin D. Das Sonnenhormon für unsere Gesundheit und der Schlüssel zur Prävention 2. Aufl. Schlangenbad: Ges. für Medizinische Information und Prävention; 2009.

Spitzer M. Meditieren im Kopf. Nervenheilkunde. 2007;26:1079–82.

Tang Y-Y, Hölzel BK, Posner MI. The neuroscience of mindfulness meditation. Nat Rev Neurosci. 2015;16(4):213–25.

Tankou SK, Regev K, Healy BC, et al. A probiotic modulates the microbiome and immunity in multiple sclerosis. Ann Neurol. 2018;83(6):1147–61.

Thompson AJ, Banwell BL, Barkhof F, et al. Diagnosis of multiple sclerosis: 2017 revisions of the McDonald criteria. Lancet Neurol. 2018;17(2):162–73.

Topping DL, Clifton PM. Short-chain fatty acids and human colonic function: role of resistant Starch and nonstarch polysaccharides. Physiol Rev. 2001;81:1031–64.

Tumani H, Petereit HF, Gerritzen A, Groß CC, Huss A, et al. S1-Leitlinie: Lumbalpunktion und Liquordiagnostik. DGNeurologie. 2019;2(6):456–80.

Turnbaugh PJ, Ridaura VK, Faith JJ, Rey FE, Knight R, Gordon JI. The Effect of diet on the human gut microbiome: a metagenomic analysis in humanized gnotobiotic mice. Sci Transl Med. 2009;1(6):6ra14.

Vieth R. Vitamin D supplementation, 25-hydroxyvitamin D concentrations and safety. Am J Clin Nutr. 1999;69(5):842–56.

Vieth R. Why the minimum desirable serum 25-hydroxyvitamin D level should be 75 mol/L (30ng/ml). Best Pract Res Clin Endocrinol Metab. 2011;25(4):681–91.

Wagner T, et al. Bundesgesundheitsbl. 2019;62:494–515.

Wallin MT, Culpepper WJ, Nicols E, et al. GDB 2016 Multiple Sclerosis Collaborators. Global, regional and national burden of multiple sclerosis 1990-2016. Lancet Neurol. 2019;18(3):269–85.

Wang Y, Marling SJ, Mc Knight SM, Danielson AL, Severson KS, Deluca HE. Suppression of experimental autoimmune encephalomyelitis by 300-315 nm ultraviolet light. Arch Biochem Biophys. 2013;536(1):81–6.

Wattjes M, Raab P. Zerebrale und spinale Bildgebung der Multiplen Sklerose: ein update. Akt Neurol. 2018;45:29–43.

Weidemann ML, Ziemssen T. Multiple Sklerose-Krankheit der 1000 Gesichter. Kompendium ZNS. 2019;1:32–8.

Wildemann B, Oschmann P, Reiber H. Neurologische Labordiagnostik. Stuttgart: Thieme Verlag; 2006.

Winek K, Dirnagl U, Meisel A. Die Deutung des intestinalen Mikrobioms beim ischämischen Schlaganfall. Akt Neurol. 2018;45:127–34.

Worm N. Heilkraft D: Wie das Sonnenvitamin vor Herzinfarkt. Krebs und anderen Zivilisationskrankheiten schützt: Systemed Verlag; 2009.

Wu Y, Benjamin EJ, MacMahon S. Prevention and control of cardiovascular disease in the rapidly changing economy of China. Circulation. 2016;133(24):2545–60.

Wunsch M, Jabari S, et al. The enteric nervous system is a potential autoimmune target in multiple sclerosis. Acta Neuropathol. 2017;134(2):281–95.

Zeng Q, Junli G, Liu X, et al. Gut dysbiosis and lack of short chain fatty acids in a Chinese cohort of patients with multiple sclerosis. Neurochem Int. 2019;129:104469.

Zettl U. Impfungen gegen Infektionskrankheiten bei Multiple Sklerose. Nervenheilkunde. 2020;39:162–6.

Index

© The Editor(s) (if applicable) and The Author(s), under exclusive license to Springer-Verlag
GmbH, DE, part of Springer Nature 2023
A. Friedrich, *The Multiple Sclerosis Companion*, https://doi.org/10.1007/978-3-662-67540-3